A
Time To L

Vivienne Tsouris

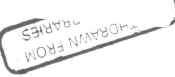

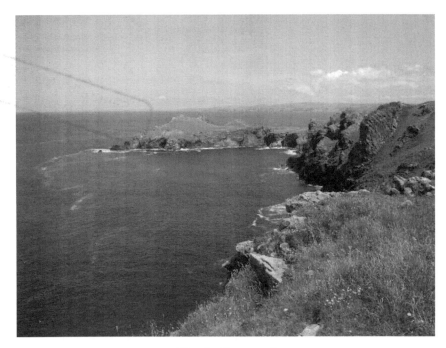

North Cornwall

A
Time To Dance

Vivienne Tsouris

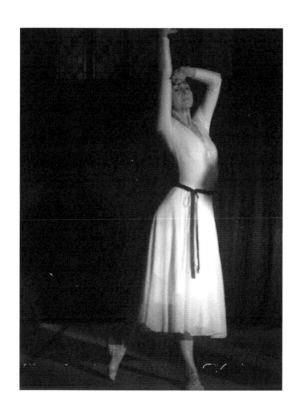

First published 2008

© Copyright Vivienne Tsouris 2008

Published by Vivienne Tsouris

ISBN 978-0-9560674

Typeset in Baskerville
Printed and bound in Great Britain by The Short Run Press, Exeter.
Design, layout Dimitris Tsouris
Cover and internal photography Jude Tsouris
Additional photography June Janes and archival sources

All poems by Vivienne Tsouris

A TIME TO DANCE

In memory of my parents
William James and May Lillian Nicholls

'Earth is crammed with heaven
and every common bush afire with God.
But only he who sees takes off
his shoes'

Elizabeth Barrett-Browning

Contents

.

'The time that I saw Vivienne perform made an impression on me. Being a musician, I probably look for other qualities in a performance than dancers do. To see profound communication and experience on stage is what makes me look and listen. To me Vivienne is a communicator'.
Nina Åström. Singer-songwriter, musician. Star of TV and radio. Represented Finland in The Eurovision Song Contest in Stockholm in 2000.

'Vivienne dances with passion and intensity, as well as with great skill and grace. Yet in a way her dance is meditative: her movements often convey a quiet, deeply rooted faith, for they seem to emanate from an inner core of certainty that she is held by a gracious loving God'.
Geoffrey Stevenson. Actor and mime artist. Founding member of Riding Lights Theatre Company.

'Vivienne has performed often at our annual Christian Artists Seminars in The Netherlands. We have seen that hard work, focus, and an open mind are the basics for excellence. Vivienne has been an ambassador for these attitudes. She is a great example of the power to overcome many hindrances in personal, professional and public life. Vivienne has excellent teaching abilities and is able to work with participants of all ages'.
Leen & Ria La Rivière
Directors. International Association of Christian Artists, Rotterdam, The Netherlands. Leen La Rivière is author of 22 books about the arts and culture. He is Chairman of the CNV Kunstenbond (the Christian National Trade Union for Artists), The National Council of Music (of the Netherlands), Continental Ministries Europe and Director of The Continental Art Centre, Rotterdam.

'As the Cathedral lights were dimmed, Vivienne Tsouris, a lithe and elegant white-clad dancer, moved down the length of the nave. This graceful young woman's lissom and expressive interpretation of Michael Neil's music has completely won me round to a proper appreciation of liturgical dance'.
Sue Cotton
A See of Lights: Truro Cathedral 2002

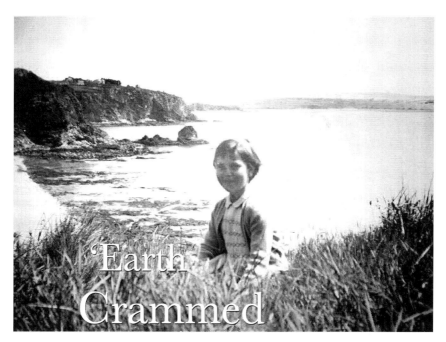

'Earth Crammed

with Heaven'

In the restless, ceaselessly undulant ocean of life, little islands of memory somehow crystallize; tiny fragments caught forever in the mind's eye. Pictures, strangely redolent of hazy, bygone days, but which at any moment are capable of sparking into life a myriad of magical, sensory recollections.

The curved white clouds suspended in the vast sky, like so many circus animals and clowns in joyful procession. The vibrancy of the garden peonies as they burst forth from their tight buds into an extravagance of vivid red petals, creating cool exotic caverns for exploring insects.

And how evocative the smells! Whether the fragrance of primroses as they peeped through the hedgerows, or the pungent aroma of marshland with its succulent foliage, or less enchanting perhaps, but equally memorable, the mustiness of wooden desks and classrooms at the beginning of each new school term. The sinking feeling of hopeless resignation which accompanied that particular smell, mingled with the unfamiliarity and stiffness of gymslip, blazer and squeaky new shoes.

Worst of all were the fears. So dominating as they invaded my young life! The concrete-textured bears, phantom residue of an earlier nightmare, were monsters which, in spite of their solid and supposedly restrictive anatomy, apparently found no difficulty whatsoever in prowling the dark corridors of human habitation, devouring with great delight all foolishly unsuspecting children. And the long, whispering wraiths that haunted the shadows, or stood like sentinels, partially concealed behind the curtains; patiently, diligently, observing my every move. I would lie in bed at night, watching them as they peeped at me from behind the bedroom door, waiting for me to fall asleep. These silent, nameless beings gradually came to dominate and control almost every moment of my waking hours.

Stored somewhere, deep within the treasure trove of my mind, are scores of these prism-like gems of memory; tiny fragments of isolated incidents, many of which occurred sometime during the summer of 1948. All are strung together by an invisible thread, and held for a lifetime, indelibly imprinted within the pathways of that miraculous storehouse, the human brain.

My parents had moved from suburban Enfield shortly after the war, and undertaken the running of a large guest-house at Bigbury-on-Sea. This particular stretch of the South Devon coastline is undeniably beautiful, but the waters, especially around the Bigbury area, are renowned for their treacherous unpredictability. There were frequent, tragic drownings in the bay close to our house. The anxiety of endeavouring to combine business with caring for her four children must have weighed heavily upon my mother, not least because my two brothers, aged six and twelve years, were both wildly keen to explore this exciting new world of cliffs, caves, islands and whirlpools.

At two years old, I was more interested in carrying out my investigations closer to the security of home. This is not an age when one is apt to consider the consequences of one's misdemeanours. The sight of a huge, thick, yellow blancmange, which had undoubtedly been prepared with great care as a dessert for the unsuspecting guests, presented an unparalleled opportunity for research. My small fingers were inserted and came out tasting quite delicious, but still more intriguing were the little holes that subsequently appeared in the pudding.

"How did this happen?" My mother exclaimed later that day when the crime was discovered. "Why, there must have been a little mouse in the kitchen!" I said nothing, and felt not the slightest compunction at casting the blame for my transgressions upon any other living soul, least of all an anonymous rodent.

In a large wooden trunk in the hall, lay a life-sized china doll whose name was Shirley, a much prized possession of my sister's. In a previous existence this doll had spent its days reclining languidly in shop windows, gazing out upon busy London streets, arrayed in a constantly changing variety of fashionable attire, as is the lot of all mannequins. I was both fascinated and horrified by this lifeless, blond-haired beauty, who now lay motionless in her coffin-like resting place, and who stared up at me out of glassy blue eyes whenever I ventured to peep beneath the lid. I do not remember doing so, but apparently it was I who was responsible for inflicting this death-like state upon the doll. I had attempted to raise her giant form into my arms, and in the process had accidentally cracked her brittle limbs. There she lay in all her ghastly beauty, a silent but indisputable testimony to my guilt.

Like our forefathers of Eden, temptation was not something I gave a great deal of resistance to during those early years. Or perhaps it was more a case of curiosity. For example, was it possible that this large, juicy blackberry might just fit the cavity of my right nostril? I clearly recall my attempt to find out. And yes, it did………perfectly! However, the obstruction refused to budge afterwards, and it took my father's resourcefulness, combined with liberal amounts of pepper, to remove the offending blockage.

"I tished, and it cummed out!" I explained to all and sundry after this interesting episode of personal experiment.

Adults, furniture, playthings such as the rocking horse, or my brother's bicycle, were all immensely tall and of strange dimensions. My father's wellington boots created a wondrous impression upon me as he stood, towering beside me, precariously straddled across a stream, gathering watercress. I remember crying to be carried along the beach by my giant-sized, elongated sister, who has since shrunk to similar proportions as myself, at around five feet four inches.

Colouring-in was a revelatory experience. No matter how hard I pressed, the yellow crayon staunchly refused to make any notable impression upon the white surface of my drawing pad. Once I was given a wonderful new pencil, with a different coloured tip at each end. I recall the excitement as I anticipated the possibility of being able to draw with both colours simultaneously. And then the frustration at discovering that science just wasn't on my side!

Aeons later (for such seemed the passing of a single year in those days), my family was on the move again, this time to the little Cornish hamlet of Tregorrick, about a mile from St. Austell town. It must have been springtime when we went to view the tiny cottage that was to become our home for the next three years, for I was entranced by the purple, primrose-like flowers that grew along the garden path. I can never look at these particular flowers now without feeling that same stab of wonder, like catching at the threads of a dream from another world, just as it slips away.

There was a big girl called Jean Rowden who lived just down the lane from us, in a tiny ramshackle cottage. Jean liked to play with me, taking me under her wing in a motherly fashion. Mr. Rowden grew the most amazing flowers in his garden: roses, sweet peas, gladioli, dahlias, lilies; blossoms of every imaginable shape, size and colour. He frequently sent my brother and me home bearing wonderfully fragrant bouquets to present to our Mum. His wife liked to talk to my mother about all the 'goings-on' in the neighbourhood. She had a habit of uttering, in a hushed, scarcely audible voice, what she clearly considered to be the most shocking bits of gossip, and then, closing her eyes and turning her back on her listener, she would walk away some six feet or so, as if in demonstration of the fact that she was so appalled by what she had just revealed that she had lost the power of speech and needed to go home to recuperate. Her disability rarely lasted more than ten seconds, however, after which time she invariably made a swift and complete recovery.

I was the only little girl living in the village at this time. My brother, Graham, being four years older than I, was incredibly patient and protective of me, often allowing me to accompany him and his playmates on their treks through Bluebell Wood, or across the fields and marshes where we played cowboys and Indians, or made secret camps. Whenever these missions were considered excessively hazardous, necessitating the boys' venturing further afield, I would be gently persuaded to stay at home and amuse myself, which I was usually quite happy to do. We had a swing suspended from an elder tree in one corner of the garden, and I used to sit there, dangling from the rope, playing 'Dying Day'. The concept of dying fascinated me but I thought everybody had to do it at the same time. Maybe this was an innate sense of The Final Judgement, or perhaps I was just mistaken.

Jean Rowden took me along to Sunday school once, but I was just too shy to cope with such exposure. God was ok, but I couldn't handle all the people and the unfamiliar surroundings. There was one sunny, breezy morning when, without a care in the world, I followed my Mum out into the garden to watch her hang the washing on the line. For a while I became engrossed in an imaginary discovery of fairies amongst the foliage. Then dawned the awful realization that my mother had disappeared indoors, leaving me defenseless in this frightening expanse of jungle! Looking up at the sky I noticed, for the first time, giant sinister-looking clouds hovering ominously above me. Fear gripped my heart as I recalled the account of Christ's ascension in my Children's Picture Bible. '.........*And a cloud came down from Heaven and received him out of their sight.*' Panic-stricken, I took to my heels and dashed indoors lest I, too, should be whisked away and likewise transported to Paradise!

These were the days when the sun seemed always to be shining, especially at weekends. But I do recall one very rainy day, and it happened to be a Sunday. I bounced out of bed, looked out of the window and found, to my utter surprise, little rivulets running down the garden path. I stomped downstairs and questioned my all-knowing Dad about the discrepancy.

"It shouldn't rain today," I complained. "It's Sunday. Why is it called Sunday if there's no sun?"

Well, you learn something new every day! But maybe the sun did put in an appearance by the time the familiar smell of roast beef and Yorkshire pudding began to mingle with Family Favourites on the wireless. Then the little man who lived inside it would announce, "This is the British Forces Network in Germany." And the theme tune, 'There's a Song in My Heart' floated gently through the atmosphere, and seemed to alight like a sprinkling of sugar upon my Mum's home-made apple pie.

With the advent of my fifth birthday I was, so they told me, ready to start school. Being an agonizingly shy child, I initially found it a terrifying place. My concerned parents attempted to alleviate my distress by sending me to a small private school, which probably prevented me from dying of shock on the first day. I remember accompanying my mother on a guided tour around the premises, prior to my being taken on as a pupil. Mr. Dorman, the head-teacher, mentioned that the school colours were brown and green. This mystified me as the main building was of grey stone, admittedly with green guttering, and the gymnasium and hut-like classrooms that were dotted around the playground were all painted with creosote.

A few weeks later, dressed in my crisp white blouse, my brown gymslip and hat with the green badge stitched to its wide brim, I followed my Mum unsuspectingly through the school gates. Little did I know that a virtual eternity of full-time education lay ahead of me! But my main task right now was one of survival on a daily basis. Fortunately I was collected at lunchtime when I was taken home, fed, and bolstered with encouragement before being deposited once again at my little wooden desk. In spite of my timid disposition, I was chosen for the part of Mary in my first nativity play. I uttered not a word but sat by the crib, trying unsuccessfully not to beam with pleasure as my classmates made their entrances and exits dressed as angels, shepherds, wise men, sheep, cows and donkeys; all bearing gifts for my baby doll whom I tenderly rocked in its little wicker cradle.

I remained in Kindergarten throughout my first two terms, after which I was moved into Transition, where my teacher, Miss Trudgett, taught us 'twystymes'. After much struggling and heartache, I was at last able to timidly join my classmates in the monotonous recitation of this mysterious chant. Then, would you believe it! Miss Trudgett had the audacity to leave. A new teacher turned up and blew the whole thing apart by declaring twystymes redundant and introducing entirely foreign lyrics.......'One two is two, two twos are four' and so on. I was devastated!

For some unaccountable reason my sixth birthday stands out in my memory above all others. I had a pretty card that pictured fairies dancing along blades of grass, and a beautifully illustrated book called Pookie and the Gypsies (Pookie was a white rabbit who had successfully mastered the powers of flight). I piled all my presents onto my splendid new basket chair and carried them up to show Barrie, my elder brother, who was ill in bed at the time. Taking his sickness into consideration, I probably felt it safe to take this risk. Under normal circumstances I might well have been in danger of death by tickling, or at least be subjected to merciless teasing.

"Shut your eyes and open your mouth, and see what God will send you," he would say sweetly. Obediently I stood with eyes screwed up, tongue protruding, awaiting the heavenly gift...only to be blessed with a mouthful of mustard!

Being a musician, Barrie was actually to become a tremendous influence on me artistically. Thanks to the fact that the personal stereo had yet to be invented, our whole family had no choice but to be immersed in the music of Bessie Smith, Louis Armstrong, Mahalia Jackson and a whole host of artists whose richness and powerful, earthy qualities would often leave me close to tears, and bursting with an unidentified longing for creative expression.

Evidently my seventh year was significant in that it made a lasting impression on me. Christmas 1952 remains with me still. I sensed a certain secrecy regarding some aspects of the festive season, which were not, however, sufficiently disturbing to cause me to probe further into the enigma. In addition to two baby dolls, Santa Claus had also left a beautiful new pram. How strange, then, that on more than one occasion I distinctly overheard my mother refer to it as my sister's dolls-pram with a fresh coat of paint!

✦ ✦ ✦ ✦ ✦ ✦ ✦ ✦ ✦ ✦ ✦ ✦ ✦

I am so grateful that I had the privilege of growing up as a member of a fair-sized family, before community life was all but obliterated by the over-use of the car, and homes came to be dominated by the presence of TV. My parents together formed a solid rock of security as unshakable as the world itself, and instilled within me a sense of profound worth. All children should have the right to grow up with the understanding that they are special. After all, we are *'fearfully and wonderfully made'*, (1) each with incredible potential. Problems only arise when one of us develops the idea that we are more special than the rest! I remember being much impressed when my mother assured me that she would never part with me. No, not for all the money in the world! Of course, I had never really suspected she would, but it seemed to me to emphasize for the first time, the worthlessness of material possessions when compared to the value of human relationships.

Whilst my mother was the embodiment of common sense, my father was the very epitome of omniscience and wisdom. I remember the day he confessed to me, having first been closely questioned on the matter, that he didn't actually understand or know about everything in the world. I'm not sure I believed him!

Diana, my sister, being more than fourteen years my senior, was like a second mother to me, and I loved her as such. It seemed that I always had an adult on hand for extra protection and extra treats. I liked her to take me on walks, and for days out at the seaside. I also have happy memories of her reading to my brother and me, cosily ensconced beside the log fire on winter evenings. She was rather like a princess, being very pretty and kind. Besides, she used to dress up in high-heeled shoes and rustling skirts of taffeta, and go to dances. Sometimes she even brought me home streamers, or balloons, from these magical-sounding events.

Barrie, ten years my senior, always seemed grown-up to me. Apart from his musical influence upon the family, his chief role has been making us all laugh. I can never remember him being grumpy or miserable. He was an accomplished teaser, and thanks to his constant provocations I eventually learnt the wisdom of not rising to take the bait, a valuable lesson in life. He always knew exactly how to wind people up. I can see my Mum now, cowering in the kitchen, simultaneously shrieking and laughing, with Barrie growling ominously and brandishing the blunt side of the carving knife!

My childhood hero was, of course, Graham, although I was not consciously aware of our closeness at the time. He was a tower strength and protection to me, particularly outside the home. Yet nobody, but nobody, could ever be told about the long, shadowy wraiths who came to dominate my young life with ever-increasing tyranny!

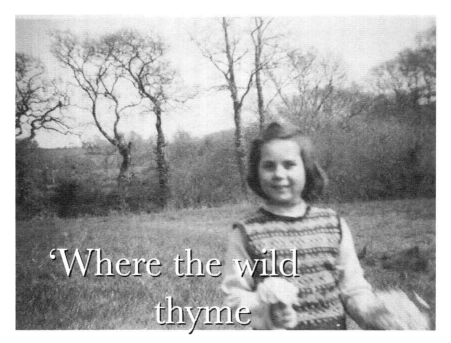

'Where the wild thyme blows'

In the spring of 1953 my parents bought 'Byways', the cottage next door, along with a disused Sunday school hall which adjoined it. Once the necessary alterations had been completed, this afforded us the luxury of much needed extra space, the previous cottage having been so small. The Big Room, as the converted Sunday school became known, was a wonderful place for family parties, and was well able to accommodate Barrie's new Première drum kit, much to the annoyance of some of our more grumpy neighbours. In all fairness, I think it was only Maude who was particularly adversely affected. Maude was a skinny, sour-faced, apron-clad charwoman with a crabby temper. I remember her complaining bitterly to the congregation of cats that constantly swarmed about her, "He just bangs away on they-there drums all day. It wouldn't be so bad if he could play a tune!" Maude worked as a daily help for Old Mrs. George, who lived opposite us. She clearly had a huge chip on her shoulder and was exceedingly pessimistic. She resented the existence of all children, and vehemently accused the world of starving its entire cat population.

The comparative spaciousness of our new home inspired my mother to open the place to summer visitors, and a large B&B sign was erected at the bottom of the hill, by the Tregorrick turning. In the garden stood two somewhat dilapidated stone sheds which, once they had been knocked together, extended, and had become the subject of a complete redecorating programme, were grandly renamed 'The Chalet'. Here our family resided during the summer months whilst my poor old Mum spent hours tending to the needs of the holidaymakers who took over our rooms.

I found this annual exodus quite exciting; rather like camping, but with the additional comfort of a slate roof and solid floor. It was one summer day, whilst we were resident in The Chalet, that my father called me out into the early morning sunshine to watch the dew falling; a phenomenon I have never witnessed since.

While my mother prepared breakfast for the visitors, I would make my daily pilgrimage, wandering alone across the fields to the marshes, where the sunlight made rainbows as it shone through the morning mist that hung over the reeds and spiders' webs. Mr. George's farm stood nearby. In his friendly manner he would often chat to me, inviting me into the farmyard to see the animals, and perhaps take a look at his newest calf.

Mr. and Mrs. George and their two sons, Angus and Adrian, who were also our playmates, lived in a large house named Bridgemead, so-called because it overlooked the fields which led down to the little iron bridge that crossed the white clay-river, far away at the bottom of the hill. Mistakenly, I thought their house-name was Bridge–Meat, since they ran a butcher's shop in their garden. The Georges also owned an orchard from which all the children in the neighbourhood scrumped vast amounts of apples. Little did we realize that this good-natured couple knew all about our acts of criminality, as we stood, just outside the orchard, pockets and cheeks bulging, waving sheepishly as they trundled past in their old car.

There were three working farms in Tregorrick during the fifties. This was just prior to the advent of mechanization, which largely put an end to our ancient farming traditions. Looking back, one realizes how privileged our generation was to be involved in such age-old customs as hay-making and the corn harvest, which were then still accomplished with the aid of horse and plough. In June, when the weather was hot and the grass high, the entire male contingent of the village rallied together and worked around the clock in a concerted effort to make and gather hay while favourable conditions prevailed. Without the aid of the tractor, the local farmers were reliant solely upon manpower and their carthorses.

Initially the grass was cut and left to dry out for a day or two. We youngsters were then encouraged to romp and play in the fields, tossing and turning the drying grasses. A few days later the real work began. Graham was among the group of small boys who joined forces with the men of the village on these occasions. The adults, armed with pikes, and the children with their bare hands, gathered the hay and helped carry it to the hay-cart, to which Prince, the enormous cart-horse, stood patiently harnessed. Mr. George's farmhand, Harry Stark, arranged the hay as it was hoisted aloft the wagon by the other workers.

At lunchtime, Mrs. George would appear with a wicker basket, covered with a white linen cloth, and filled with hot pasties, saffron cake, and other homemade treats. The men and boys, hot and thirsty after their hard work, took a welcome rest whilst this wonderful village picnic was spread before them in the field. Jugs of tea were brought, together with bottles of skit, a kind of traditional lemonade which had been prepared by Old Mrs. George, especially for the children.

Throughout the day, Prince dutifully transported each brimming cartload of hay along the lanes to the open barn, where the rick was to be constructed; a job that required Harry's expertise. The villagers gathered the hay onto their pikes and passed it up to him as he built the rick, all the time rising higher and higher as the mountain of hay grew beneath his feet.

One year Prince was bitten by a horsefly. To everyone's horror, he reacted by bolting from the scene of toil while still harnessed to the hay-cart, which was full, almost to capacity. Horse and cart went careering through the lanes at a frenzied gallop, allegedly with one small boy still clinging to the reigns. Amazingly, nobody was hurt!

In August, when the corn was ripe and ready for harvesting, the villagers once again prepared to lend a helping hand. This time the children's job was to arrange the sheaves of corn into stooks, which were then left to stand in the fields for a couple of days, to allow the grains to dry out. Finally, the stooks were gathered up and carried to the thresher. I was too small to be of any use on these occasions, but for many of Tregorrick's youngsters, these long summer days were filled from morning till night with pure enchantment and delight.

++++++++++++++

Apart from our house-move, 1953 was also a notable year nationally. I was much more happily settled at school by this time, and at seven years old had graduated to the first form. One very special day we were treated to a showing of a technicolour film about Sir Edmund Hilary's recent conquest of Everest. This was also the year of the coronation, and, as TV culture had not yet thrust itself upon us to the detriment of community life, our entire school was taken to see this on film, at the local cinema.

I remember well the day of the coronation itself, and all the local celebrations. These took place in the tiny, neighbouring village of London Apprentice. It was a fine June day and for some unaccountable reason I won first prize in several races, each time being rewarded with a shiny sixpence. Ever since that day I have maintained a steady reputation for being useless at all sports activities, although I did manage to win the high jump cup one year at the inter-school sports.

In fact, the arrival of our annual sports day heralded a time of silent agonizing for me. Because our school had no sports field of its own, we used facilities at the opposite end of town. These lay on the far side of the town park, beyond which I had to navigate my way through several meandering gardens and some tennis courts, before arriving at my destination. The prospect of losing my way in this alien landscape filled me with trepidation. I had a cunning strategy whereby I supposedly set off for school on the dreaded day, but secretly made a detour around the lanes and ended up hiding in a field until the coast was clear. The field was full of feverfew plants, and to this day the scent of this daisy-like flower never fails to induce in me feelings of guilt and anxiety. I still struggle with this same problem of geographical incompetence. I am convinced that I was born with a vital deficiency of the brain which has rendered me void of any sense of direction.

My inability to find my way about, together with my timidity, caused me to suffer an enormous sense of inferiority and inadequacy, which prohibited me from venturing on school outings. While other children thronged excitedly to see puppet shows, or visited museums or attended concerts, I stayed behind, safe and secure in my classroom, busily engaging in mathematical problems or writing essays. Years later, during my final year at school in Cornwall, I somehow summoned up the courage to accompany my classmates on an educational trip to Truro, culminating in a guided tour around the cathedral. I loved every minute of it and found the cathedral especially fascinating. Little did I think that some forty years hence, I would be dancing down that enormous aisle by candlelight, before many hundreds of people, symbolizing, in my white dress, the light of the world, as the Celtic saints of old introduced the gospel of Christ to the pagan communities of ancient Cornwall. But all this is, as yet, far, far into the future!

✝ ✝ ✝ ✝ ✝ ✝ ✝ ✝ ✝ ✝ ✝ ✝

I have a sneaking suspicion that I was the only child of my day who was constantly scolded for being too quiet. A proper stick-in-the-mud! My mother worried that I was abnormal, and her anxiety was probably quite justified. Next to my parents, the person with the greatest influence upon me was Graham, my brother closest to me in age. He was something of a philosopher, and in his kind, gentle way he began to open my eyes to the beauty of nature, and the unspoilt world around us. Gradually, intuitively, I became aware of the age-old paradox: that beauty and suffering go hand in hand. And as the world confronted me with its unfathomable mixture of heartache and loveliness, I would sit idly daydreaming, lost in thought. Or maybe wander through the country lanes, contemplating the miracle of every living thing that popped out at me as I ambled along, weaving stories of fairyland in and through the stem of each flower that I clutched in my grubby little hand. To talk about trivialities seemed a futile exercise, not worth wasting breath over. However, I secretly longed to be accomplished, like most other people, in the art of small talk, and frequently marvelled at the predictability of their comments.

Gradually, with every passing year, the world took on a paler hue; still crammed with heaven's mysteries, but less intensely so. Yet this was a golden time. As the seasons changed, so we children were absorbed into the magical transformation of the woods and fields around us, for in those days the world was filled with magic. The soft, dark, leafy soil that constituted the floor of our secret camp, among the rhodedendrons in the bluebell wood. The brush of the tall ferns and bracken against our bare legs as we pushed our way through the undergrowth, towards the pond, into which at least one of our number would inevitably fall during the course of the day. The fat, heavy drops of summer rain as they beat upon the broad leaves of the sycamore tree, under whose ample boughs we sheltered. The sad sight of a dead bird by the hedge; or those gripping, anxious moments, as one crouched close to the earth, breathing in the sweet scents of foliage, moss and decaying leaves; heart racing, hoping against hope to outwit the other players in a game of hide-and-seek. All these simple pleasures filled the long days of our childhood. Now we walk upon the surface of the earth, but in those carefree times we were a part of its very breath, its rhythm and its substance.

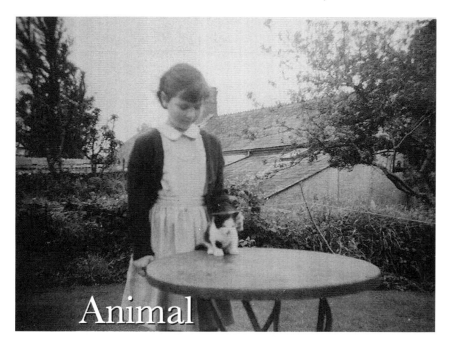

Animal Crackers

One of the nicest aspects of being the youngest child in the family is that the older siblings eventually bring home all manner of friends, and a great deal of fun can be had by simply 'showing off'. I was undoubtedly a complete nuisance, but Diana's boyfriends, and later, Barrie's young ladies, were all admirably tolerant of me, and I considered them to be my greatest friends.

In 1956 I had the immense joy of being chief bridesmaid at my sister's wedding, and the following December I acquired the impressive title of 'Auntie' when her son, Nicholas, was born. I was unspeakably proud of my new nephew and totally prejudiced against all other babies. These I regarded, without exception, as being quite inferior to this beloved child whom I loved, and will always love, as my own brother. During the same year Barrie left home to do his national service in the army. I missed him so much. There was nobody to tease me; no one to drive me to distraction by claiming to be prettier than our pet budgerigar. I used to send him parcels of sweets: licorice bootlaces, sugar mice, parma violets and chewing gum. I felt so sorry for him.

I loved animals, and my first experience of real sorrow was when the unfortunate budgie was discovered lying, feet uppermost, at the bottom of its cage. I bought a little mouse which very soon suffered a similar fate. In my grief I vowed I would never bury her, but keep her in a matchbox so that I could continue to look at her and stroke her silky brown coat. A few days later, I opened the box for my daily devotional contemplation of my little pet, only to find that she had been transformed into a mass of crawling maggots! Sentimentality went out of the window, along with the remains of my beloved mouse!

We had four she-cats which produced endless amounts of kittens. It was a relief when a pet-shop opened in town and we were able to offer an unlimited supply of small cats. I used to play with them like dolls, knitting dresses for them, wheeling them about in my dolls-pram, and training them for such prodigious occasions as the Tregorrick Circus. This epic event was produced, directed and performed by Yours Truly, and was held in the garden of Byways. The only trick at which I was reasonably accomplished was juggling. This I could do easily using three balls, and with considerable irregularity using four. I also performed a dance on a pair of stilts, which my father had made for my birthday, to the song Never Smile at a Crocodile. But as there was no music, the audience was called upon either to sing along or else use liberal amounts of imagination.

During the trapeze act, which was performed on my swing (more imagination required), I bumped my head and dissolved into tears of embarrassment. Muffled laughter could be heard coming from the auditorium. With deeply wounded pride, but full of professional spirit, I determined that the show must go on.

This circus preceded modern-day regulations restricting the use of animals for public performances. We had lions and tigers! Graham, my stage-manager, had kindly supplied a log and a plank of wood for the construction of a primitive seesaw. Three small kittens were placed on the lower end of the plank. Then, with an imaginary roll on the drums, Mother Cat was ceremoniously dropped onto the raised end. All three kittens immediately flew into the air, turned somersaults, and landed back on their feet! Amazing!!!

My sister's husband, a strapping fellow of six feet two with muscles to match, was called upon to perform the humiliating act of the strong man who was incapable of lifting our fiendishly realistic set of cardboard cut-out weights. At this point Graham and I appeared as stagehands, scooping up the hitherto impossibly heavy weights with nonchalant ease and tossing them casually backstage.

However, the pièce de résistance of the entire show was Petronella, The Performing Pigeon. Petronella was a young pigeon which Graham had once found with a bullet hole through its crop. He had brought it home, sewn it up with needle and cotton, and nursed it back to health. (It was customary for the people of Tregorrick to bring any sick or injured birds to Graham, should they happen to find any). By the time Petronella had fully recovered, her homing instincts had got the better of her and she refused to be set free. She was happy to take a quick fly around the garden, but always returned home after these brief excursions.

On the day of the circus, when Petronella was scheduled to make her début, she was brought out of the aviary with great pomp and ordered to perform. I had no idea what I expected her to do, and in retrospect, neither did she. She perched on my hand for a few moments, quizzically eyeing her audience. Suddenly, she seemed to sense some deeper instinct surging through her little pigeon brain......... the call to freedom! Petronella flew joyfully over the garden hedge never to return!

In spite of this anti-climax, the circus was generally considered a great success. I was even presented with a beautiful bouquet of flowers by Monica Snell, a young woman who lived at the bottom of the hill, in a cottage with a nice garden. Certainly everyone seemed to have enjoyed themselves...... except possibly the cats!

✦ ✦ ✦ ✦ ✦ ✦ ✦ ✦ ✦ ✦ ✦ ✦

As one might conclude from these anecdotes, animals played a big part in my life as a child. My best friend was a Dutch rabbit named Pookie (unfortunately not of the flying variety) who was so tame he would lick my legs and come when he was called. I was also the proud owner of twenty-eight white mice (there were only two to start with!) who lived in the bird-shed with Graham's canaries.

One day, Graham turned up with a large, sandy-coloured mongrel dog from a rescue centre. I don't think my Mum was too thrilled by this unexpected addition to the family, but since the only alternative was that the poor animal should be put down, she relented, much to our delight. The dog's name was Susie and she obviously considered her main mission in life was to bark as long and as loudly as possible, which is probably why she had come so perilously close to extinction.

The long-suffering cats were frequently the honoured guests at each other's birthday parties. I had learnt to knit at an early age and liked to practise this skill by fashioning elegant party dresses for my feline friends. On my way home from school I would visit the sweet shop. Then, resisting the temptation to eat all my purchases at once, I would rush home and arrange a special tea party, using my dolls' tea set. Later that evening our entire family would be summoned into The Big Room ......the cats also being lured in unsuspectingly, with bits of bacon rind and other appropriate scraps. Out came the party clothes, and the sullen-looking cats were solemnly instructed to keep still whilst they were dressed for the occasion. One by one each animal struggled and fizzed angrily, then dashed out of the room in a shameful exhibition of ingratitude. That episode over, all the remaining guests sat and nibbled pieces of honeycomb-crunch, chocolate raisins and licorice pipes from tiny china plates, and pretended to drink the lemonade that I had prepared earlier in miniature teacups of variable states of cleanliness.

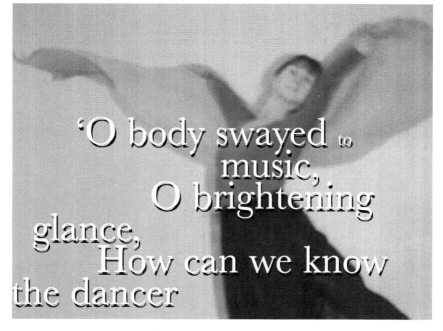

'O body swayed to music,
O brightening glance,
How can we know the dancer

from the dance?'

William Butler Yates

The stories of Hans Christian Anderson have always filled me with a combination of fascination and horror. Particularly disturbing is the concept of inanimate objects being capable of experiencing emotions such as desire, sorrow or pain, in which case these unfortunate 'beings' would all too frequently find themselves destined to an eternity of total misery and anguish. A painted shepherdess, now no more than a powdery scattering of broken china, swept into the bin; each tiny fragment forever doomed to ache with unfulfilled passion for a handsome tin soldier who has, himself, been reduced to a shapeless, though fully conscious blob of cold metal, following a fall into a blazing coal fire.

Yet there is one tale in particular that, for me, is especially significant. The Red Shoes tells of a girl with a fatal fascination for a pair of red dancing slippers. Once on her feet, the shoes compel her to dance without ceasing until the poor child finally dies of exhaustion. This, I believe, is the experience of most dancers. Once captivated by the irresistible magic of dance and theatre, one's life is never quite the same again. One becomes the loyal bondservant of discipline and exercise, and never feels truly alive unless willingly subjected to their rule of tyranny.

I was first taken to ballet lessons when I was nine-and-a-half years old. I enjoyed dancing and my teacher seemed impressed with me. Miss Luke, the ballet mistress, eagerly coached me through the early grade examinations. I achieved excellent results and within a year I was dancing on pointe. I decided that when I grew up, I would follow in my mother's footsteps and become a teacher of dance. However, something happened that was to change my life!

Shortly after my eleventh birthday, Miss Luke organized a concert. It was held in a tiny local theatre, but with sufficient authenticity about it to lend a magical feel to the evening. I danced in a piece called The Pink Ballet, clad in my pink tutu and satin pointe shoes. I was taken completely by surprise! The minute the music struck up and I stepped onto the stage, I found myself consumed by some mysterious force which sent my habitual shyness fleeing into the shadows. Life and energy burst through my entire being into movement. Footlights, music, costumes, velvet curtains, darkened auditorium, and here in the midst of it all was I, caught up in this wonderful, swirling, ecstatic moment of 'the now'.

I was hooked! I began listening much more attentively to my mother's stories of how she herself had trained as a dancer; of the shows and performances she had organized and danced in, and of her experiences in London's West End, where she had watched the legendary Anna Pavlova and Vaslav Nijinsky dance.

I started collecting books about ballet and discovered, to my amazement, that to become a dancer and work in a real theatre, one didn't necessarily have to be a princess, born with pink satin pointe shoes already attached to one's feet. Perfectly ordinary people could do it, apparently, provided they were blessed with a perfectly structured anatomy and extraordinary talent. Also, in all the ballet stories I had read, the heroine invariably had large, dark, wistful eyes and a pale oval face. Mine was undeniably round and went bright red whenever I worked really hard.

My mind was made up! I was going to be a ballerina!

✛ ✛ ✛ ✛ ✛ ✛ ✛ ✛ ✛ ✛ ✛ ✛ ✛

I have always held the belief that true magic is, at least in part, that elusive, essential quality of life which, when we find it, invariably comes as a total surprise, and is so beautiful it makes us want to cry. The older we become, the more it evades us. The more we seek after it, the faster it slips through our fingertips, like a ray of sunlight, or a shadow. My great longing as a child, and still today, is to seek after those soft, yet persistent whisperings, which can so unexpectedly nudge us into a momentary awareness of an unseen world; a world from which all of life seems ultimately to draw its meaning.

I saved my 1957 summer visitors' B&B tips and bought a record of Tchaikovsky's Swan Lake. On winter evenings, whenever The Big Room was available, I would clear back the furniture, draw faces in the condensation on the window-panes, prepare the Royal Box, and dance Odette-Odile at the Royal Opera House, Covent Garden.

In summer, when the evenings were long and light, I went out onto the car park beside our house and danced all the major classical roles I had ever heard of. There is a certain wistful nostalgia about early morning and eventide alike. They seem full of mysterious moments when God himself, or perhaps an unseen company of angels, might well be watching over us.

Years later, I discovered that I really did have an audience, not with the angelic hosts, but with Mrs. Gooding's auntie! Mrs. Gooding lived with her aged aunt, whom I never actually remember having seen, except perhaps as a faint shadow at the window of Chapel House. This old converted chapel, although separated from us by a public footpath and a sizeable vegetable garden, overlooked our house, being higher up on the slope of Tregorrick Hill. In days gone by, the chapel, together with our Sunday school, had been in regular use as places of worship.

Many years after those early 'Covent Garden' performances in the car park, I happened to meet Mrs. Gooding whilst wheeling my first-born around the Tregorrick lanes. We stopped for a chat and some baby talk. My friend then went on to tell how Auntie, long since gone to glory, had regularly enquired, every summer evening, "Is the little girl out there yet?" Her niece would then escort her to a seat by an upstairs window, from whence Auntie would sit and view my performance below. This revelation made me feel so happy, and extremely privileged, that somebody really had been sharing with me, all those years ago, in the magic of dance!

Auntie eventually bequeathed the remains of an ancient tea set to me, along with a few other oddments, in recognition of the pleasure I had unwittingly given her. All that I have left today is a tiny white and gold tea plate. A fitting souvenir of my car park performances!

+ + + + + + + + + + + + +

As very young children we come, *'not in entire forgetfulness, and not in utter naked-ness, but trailing clouds of glory from God who is our home.'*(2) Unconsciously, passive-ly, experientially, with the gradual casting aside of our celestial raiment, we imbibe from the vast sea of life its sounds and substances, its colours, tastes and textures. We learn to trust, to fear, to venture; instinct and intuition being bound together during these formative years, creating a wholeness, an inte-gration between ourselves and a world in which the childlike mind sees no division between the tangible and the spiritual.

Many are the influences, seen and unseen, that shape our character traits and individual paths. Once conscious ambition takes a hold on us, our lives and energies become channelled into a specific direction. All that was absorbed experientially during those early days, we learn to assimilate, adapt and culti-vate, until we are capable of making our own mark upon the world, choosing, to some extent, the direction of our lives; perhaps fulfilling our destiny.

And so it happened that in 1959, at the age of thirteen, I was accepted into the Rambert Ballet School, in London. The school was then based at Notting Hill, in the tiny Mercury Theatre, which had been home to the Ballet Rambert when it was first formed in 1931. Marie Rambert herself had previ-ously been a member of Diaghilev's Ballets Russes, having trained under Isadora Duncan and Enrico Cecchetti. Supportive as ever, my parents made all sorts of sacrifices on my behalf, in order that this enormous transition in my life should happen as smoothly as possible. For the first couple of weeks I took lodgings in Acton, but when this proved unsatisfactory, I moved further out of the metropolis to Enfield, where my Auntie Doris kindly took me in.

The training and discipline of The Rambert School were wonderful, but the daily travelling to and from London was really not practical for such an inexperienced youngster. My mother, understandably nervous of leaving her shy little daughter to the mercy of the crowds and traffic of the great capital, put the fear of God in me. I saw murderers and kidnappers lurking in every doorway, waiting to carry me off and commit unspeakable atrocities at my expense. As time went by we began to consider other options.

It was decided that an audition should be arranged for me at The Arts Educational School in Tring, Hertfordshire, where students were able to board. This school was the training ground for The London Festival Ballet (now The English National Ballet), which Alicia Markova and Anton Dolin (two more prodigies of the impresario Diaghilev) had established in 1951, at the time of The Festival of Britain. The school, under the directorship of Grace Cone and Olive Ripman, boasted such former pupils as Gillian Lynne (dancer and choreographer of the West End musical 'Cats'), John Gilpin, Julie Andrews, and many other celebrities who have since been nurtured and cultivated within its walls.

My audition turned out to be a 'one to one' with Ivy Baker, the head of vocational studies, who enthused earnestly about my dancing and accepted me on the spot, putting my name at the top of a long list of other hopefuls.

The following January I found myself boarding the school train at Euston station, along with hundreds of exuberant, squealing, excited girls, all clad, like myself, in blue and grey uniform. Unlike these supremely confident young ladies, I was feeling slightly bewildered, my newly acquired stockings and suspender belt only adding to my sense of incongruity. My Mum stood on the platform just below me. She leaned forward to kiss me goodbye and I was startled to see her eyes suddenly fill with tears. At that moment I realized, for the very first time, exactly what was happening: my dream had come true; I was on my way to a professional ballet boarding school......and my beloved Mum was about to catch a train home in totally the opposite direction!

+ + + + + + + + + + + +

Until my initiation at The Rambert School, I had foolishly imagined that all ballet students were of a quiet, serene disposition. Not so! And if I still entertained any doubts regarding this delusion, my new schoolmates shattered them immediately. I sat quietly watching their boisterous antics, feeling mildly alarmed, until the train eventually clanked to a halt as it drew into Watford station. A member of staff appeared whose job it was to supervise us as we clambered aboard the coach that was to take us to our final destination.

At last we arrived at Tring Park. There at the end of the long secluded drive, lined on either side by magnificent woodland, stood the ancient majestic-looking Rothschild mansion, of which King Charles 2nd had once been a resident, frequently accompanied by his mistress, Nell Gwynn, a local orange seller who later made a name for herself as an actress. She still allegedly wandered the many corridors of this imposing residence, leaving orange peel outside dormitory windows on Hallowe'en; but by 1960 she had obviously run short on her stocks.

We trooped in through the main entrance and deposited our hand luggage before descending the steps which led down to the basement. In stark contrast to the grandeur of the main building, with its immensely high ceilings, its ornate marble carvings and stately wooden staircase, upon which one might easily imagine crinolined ladies elegantly ascending and descending, here all was quite grim and basic. The floor was of grey stone and the walls bare, except for the rows of brass bells which once summoned the many servants to their various duties, for long ago this area had been their humble quarters. Timidly, I followed the other girls into one of the huge dining-halls where, in due course, we were fed and watered.

After supper I was escorted up seemingly endless flights of stairs, to the many dormitories situated at the very top of the building. I had been allocated a place in a small room shared by just four other students. There was Susan, who came from Kent, Joy from Scotland, Diana from Ireland, and Helen, who was Norwegian. Together we unpacked our suitcases, other girls occasionally popping in to greet us, or to exchange tales of holiday antics.

How strange it all seemed! How small and lonely I felt! That first night I swallowed my toothpaste after cleaning my teeth, as it suddenly struck me as unladylike to spit into the wash-basin! My dorm-mates then ushered me back to our room where I received an enlightening lecture on the subject of human reproduction, along with several other, equally useful pieces of information. I discovered that I was a virgin, although I indignantly denied the allegation when first questioned on the matter……until the meaning of the word was explained to me, when I naturally fell into a state of flushed confusion. What an ignorant, dim-witted representative of the South West I must appear!

Matron poked her head around the door, announcing that it was time for 'lights out'. We were immediately plunged into total darkness. I was horrified! It had been discovered earlier that the catch on our dormitory window was in need of repair. To eliminate the resulting icy draught, heavy wooden shutters were bolted firmly across the entire window. I would gladly have shivered with hyperthermia rather than suffer the darkness which now engulfed us. At home, my Mum had always lit a little oil lamp at night. I had become so used to this dim night-light that if ever the oil had run out, as it very occasionally did, I would wake with a start the minute the flame was extinguished. Realizing my distress, Joy produced a clock with a small luminous face. She placed this high up on the mantelpiece as a visual focus for me. The single visible glow of greenish light penetrating the thick blackness, gave me an overwhelming feeling of claustrophobia.

Naturally, all this only added to my misery and homesickness. I tried so hard to be brave in the days that followed, telling myself how fortunate I was to be accepted into such a celebrated school of dance and the arts. But there was no denying that constant unbearable ache, which began as a hollow sensation in my stomach the moment the rising bell sounded, and seemed to spread throughout my entire body as the day wore on. I felt trapped, unable to do anything but sob myself to sleep night after night. Matron was kind, the teachers understanding, even the other girls were reasonably thoughtful most of the time.

About a week later, I was summoned to the head's office. Mrs. Hearn had evidently noticed my silent suffering. After much questioning I confessed the story of my night traumas. Oh joy! I was permitted to ring my parents! Matron was called, and was instructed to leave the door of the dormitory slightly ajar, so that a little light might be allowed to shine into the room. I clung to this privilege long after the window had been fixed, only relinquishing it during the summer term, by which time Susan, who slept in the bed opposite, was complaining bitterly about the light streaming into her face. So here I remained for the next two-and-a-half years, somehow managing to survive those first unbearable months of homesickness. As students we were

25

expected to work very hard, endeavouring to cram as much traditional schooling into the day as possible, in addition to three or four hours of dance training. The great advantage of boarding school is that there is no cut off point at the end of the day. We ate, slept and lived immersed in our studies, often rising early in the morning for music practice, or to darn our pointe shoes in preparation for class. I thrived under the pressure, feeling thoroughly expanded in all my faculties.

During my initial homesickness, I discovered that nibbling offered some comfort to my misery, and like so many other unhappy pupils, I developed an unhealthy attitude towards food, oscillating between excessive bingeing and strict dieting. More often than not, the diet was scheduled to start 'tomorrow'. My teachers eyed my thickening waistline disapprovingly. My dream of becoming a sylph-like ballerina was fast disappearing.

However, by the end of my second term at Tring Park I had settled down relatively happily and was slowly growing accustomed to this new way of life. And so it happened that the shy country child, who had previously spent long hours quietly daydreaming in solitude, began to receive a thorough training in the art of dance, as well as countless other invaluable lessons including, for example, how to relate to the many other pupils with whom I came into contact throughout my time at the school. Yet I longed for those rare, precious moments when I could be alone, and on Friday evenings, when our year was allowed its weekly privilege of over-dosing on TV, I would remain in my dormitory, relishing the solitude, thinking philosophical thoughts and writing my diary.

Twice during each term, 'visiting days' were arranged, when families or friends were invited to turn up early on a Sunday morning and take us out for the day. As my folks lived too far away, my Auntie Elsie and Uncle Syd used to drive over from Enfield and take me home with them. They were very kind to me and I shall always be indebted to them for making my life at school so much more bearable. Auntie Doris usually joined us, too, on these occasions. She was another kind-hearted person whose home was always open to me. Being unmarried herself she took an avid delight in all her nieces and nephews.

During my second year at Arts Ed, my dorm-mates and I planned to celebrate my fifteenth birthday by holding a midnight feast. Somehow we succeeded in bribing prefects from the year above to buy food for us from the local grocery store. (All prefects were allowed into the village during their free hours). That spring we were troubled, yet again, by a faulty catch on our dormitory window, although this was an entirely different dormitory in another wing of the school. Once again cold air came blasting into the room. To compensate, and while we were waiting for it to be fixed, matron arranged for a little heater to be installed, which we later discovered could be used to boil a kettle. We decided to utilize this asset by heating tomato soup on it.

I can't tell you how grim it is being roused out of your sleep at 12 a.m. by the ringing of an alarm clock, and then feeling duty bound to eat your way through a huge pile of goodies. However, we very quickly warmed to the idea and with much suppressed giggling I put the soup on to boil. Ballet school teaches little in the area of practical domesticity. I failed to realize that one is supposed to open the can before heating the contents. As I attacked the hot tin with a can-opener, the boiling soup spurted out all over my hand, which was immediately covered with a huge blistering burn. It was extremely painful, but yelling was out of the question. Neither was I at liberty to report the incident to Sister in surgery next morning. Fortunately the hand healed without the burn ever being detected.

The following year I was elevated, to my utter dismay, to the much honoured status of prefect. This presented me with terrifying responsibilities which I felt truly unable to cope with. In retrospect, I can't think why I was so paralyzed with fear at this seemingly daunting challenge.

As senior pupils, we were permitted to venture into the neighbouring towns at weekends. One Saturday afternoon in the summer of '62, three of my friends and I decided to hitch a lift into Berkhamstead where Cliff Richard's new film, The Young Ones, was showing. A cheery lorry driver soon pulled up alongside us, offering us a lift in his cab. Unfortunately there were only two spare seats, and try as we might the four of us just couldn't manage to squeeze into them. Our attempt at hitch-hiking having failed, we finally resorted to the bus, and so arrived at the cinema just in time for the film which, of course, we enjoyed immensely.

Next morning, in assembly, it was solemnly announced that four senior pupils had been seen hitch-hiking the previous day. I was in utter disgrace. My prefect's badge was confiscated. I was ecstatic! My joy was short-lived, however. The following day I was re-instated with total forgiveness. Once again I was forced to take up those dreaded duties for which I felt nothing but total inadequacy.

In spite of these frivolous-sounding escapades, my final year at school was a time of intensely hard work. In addition to our O'level studies, which we took very seriously in spite of having only half the amount of traditional schooling each day, I was also studying the Advanced Ballet syllabus of the Royal Academy as well as for major examinations in Intermediate Cecchetti Ballet and ISTD Modern Ballet and Stage (for which I am happy to say I received honours). We studied, and were examined, in both the syllabi of the Royal Academy of Dancing and Cecchetti, the standard of the latter being the more difficult. During my final term, Alicia Markova came to present us with our various certificates.

My friends and I habitually broke the school rules by rising at some unearthly hour of the morning and locking ourselves into the bathroom, where we revised methodically, consuming copious amounts of black coffee in our efforts to keep awake. Much nicer were the hot summer afternoons, when, in my occasional free hour I took my books into the long grass that bordered the huge garden, and burnt the backs of my legs while studying Shakespeare's Henry IVth, or acquainting myself with the life history of the frog, or the human digestive system.

At long last, in July 1962, I walked joyfully, but somewhat tearfully away down the drive of Tring Park, leaving behind me a host of well-loved teachers, matrons and friends, as well as many never-to-be-fulfilled promises of keeping in touch and vows of life-long friendship.

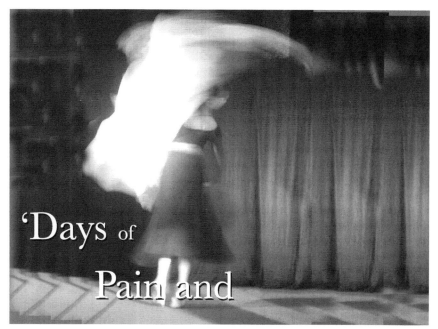

'Days of Pain and Wonder'

After much deliberating and careful consideration as to the next step in my dance training, it was decided, during one of my more rational moments (inspired, I imagine, by the news of good O'level results) that I should train as a dance teacher. Arrangements were made for me to start the following September at the Arts Educational Teacher-Training College, in London. I planned to first qualify here, before moving on to a traditional academic college of teacher-training, thereby securing two very practical strings for my bow. All the appropriate study books on technique and anatomy were purchased. My future was looking bright.

Shortly before the beginning of the new academic year I contacted Irene Luke, my Cornish ballet teacher, who had recently become an examiner with the Cecchetti Society. She was horrified by my decision, and to my secret delight, persuaded me to abandon all these sensible ideas and throw myself once more into the highly impractical pursuit of a career in the theatre. I decided to stay in Cornwall until after the New Year, taking classes with Miss Luke at her home in Newquay, since by now it was too late to arrange further auditions with London ballet schools.

The winter of 1963 was very severe, particularly in the South West. Graham attempted several bird rescuing operations, including that of a curlew whose long curved beak had frozen together, but in this instance he was unsuccessful. Eventually the train lines reopened after having been snowed under and consequently out of action for several weeks. I arrived in London on February 3rd 1963, a month late for the start of the spring term at The Andrew Hardie School of Ballet in South Kensington. At sixteen years old, living alone in a hostel in the centre of London, I felt I was quite possibly the loneliest teenager on earth. But within the space of a few weeks I settled happily into my wonderful new school (oh the joy of doing nothing but dance all day!) and before long, became good friends with a group of fellow ballet students.

The following September, three of my new chums and I moved into a bed-sitter in Onslow Gardens. In spite of our rigorous dance training we shared a fairly active social life. With Beatle mania sweeping the country, I gave up my image of the pious little ballerina who only listens to the classics, and rocked shook and twisted as vigorously as any other seventeen-year-old of that era. My friends and I became acquainted with a number of musicians who worked in well-known pop groups: Joe Brown's 'Bruvers', Georgie Fame's 'Blue Flames' and so on. We were given frequent opportunities to meet up-and-coming pop idols such as Bill Wyman of The Rolling Stones, Paul Jones, lead singer with Manfred Mann, The Who, The Shadows, as well as Arthur Brown, The God of Hellfire and folk/R&B musician, Alexis Korner.

Standing tickets for the Royal Opera House could be queued for and cost only nine shillings. The Royal Albert Hall stood just fifteen minutes walk from our bed-sit. When cheap tickets for The Proms were available, we would take our knitting (always tights or leg warmers) and spend our queuing hours clicking our needles, chattering and flirting.

That summer the Bolshoi Ballet came to London. Our entire school took turns in queuing for tickets over a period of three days. The bounty was shared equally between students and staff. I went to three of the Bolshoi's performances at the Royal Opera House, Covent Garden. The London dance scene of the day was aghast at their beauty, their strength and their amazing technical excellence. Never before had we seen such dancing! Neither had we previously witnessed the customarily regal and decorous ROH audiences behaving like soccer fans! The upper circle fairly shook with wild stamping and shouting as we broke into frenzied applause at the end of each ballet. Following this, a mad dash as we jostled through the surging crowds and out to the stage door to meet the stars and collect autographs. Vladimir Vasiliev and Ekaterina Maximova were my favourite stars. This was pure, unadulterated magic!

Looking back over my time spent as a ballet student, I think Arts Ed did an excellent job in sorting out the sheep from the goats. To be honest, I'm not sure whether the sheep were the sensible ones who, at sixteen, gave up the romantic notion of pursuing a career in dance, or vice versa. Certainly this happened in many cases. In contrast, all the students at the Andrew Hardie School were thoroughly dedicated to their work. Commitment was total. Nobody ever attempted to shirk their responsibilities or miss class.

In addition to the most excellent classical ballet training, which of course, included things like pas de deux and variation, a preparation for corps de ballet work, we were also given a daily modern dance class. This was long before contemporary dance became an established part of the curriculum of any major UK ballet school. (We students were once taken to see The Martha Graham Company when they visited London in 1964. Their power and athleticism was inspirational; and black male dancers…..well, this was quite revolutionary!) Mr. Hardie also took us for character dancing, which he himself had once studied under Lydia Sokolova. Many of the classes were open to professionals and it was always exciting when stars of the Royal Ballet, Ballet Rambert or other well-known companies appeared. Once Merle Park forgot her pointe shoes and Maggie Vickers, my flat-mate, lent her a pair, which she later autographed. I was envious, but my feet were a half size too big!

We all loved Mr Hardie, although we were greatly in awe of his often gruff manner and large stick! He had, of course, been a professional dancer himself for many years, having trained under Idzikowsky and Legat, as well as with Sokolova, all former stars of the Russian ballet. Following a highly successful career, during which he appeared in many Covent Garden productions, as well as dancing in Mona Inglesby's International Ballet, he became a teacher at the Judith Espinosa School. Finally, in 1958, he had opened his own school in South Kensington.

Andrew Hardie was, without question, one of London's best teachers of classical ballet at that time. We worked ourselves to the point of exhaustion in order to please him. Over the studio door hung a notice, 'Here we Suffer

Grief and Pain'. I owe to my beloved Mr. Hardie the ability both to continue dancing at a professional level (even into my late fifties) and also to teach the classical technique.

✦ ✦ ✦ ✦ ✦ ✦ ✦ ✦ ✦ ✦ ✦ ✦ ✦

A year lasted so long in those days! I'm sure one was able to cram a great deal more into life on account of this. In 1964 I fell in love for the first time. This had a profound effect upon me as it awakened in me a new realization: namely that my life-long ambition to dance was totally incompatible with another, previously unarticulated desire: to some day be married with a family of my own. This revelation brought me face to face with a seemingly impossible inner conflict, and was a contributing factor to my becoming ill with a nervous disorder. In spite of my relentless training programme, I found myself unable to sleep or eat properly. I suffered panic attacks when my restricted breathing caused my vision to black out, frightening me nearly to death. My head and back ached constantly. I resorted to pep pills as a means of coping with my daily classes. I felt totally exhausted. All this eventually resulted in my having to take six months out from ballet school. I was sent back to Cornwall to recuperate, armed with a collection of brightly coloured tranquilizers and sleeping pills which had been prescribed by my doctor. In those days I innocently trusted the medical profession and knew nothing of natural or alternative remedies. Now began a painful period of great inner turmoil and confusion. Much water was to pass under the bridge of time before the conflict could ever begin to resolve itself.

But Cornwall is such a wonderful place to rediscover peace and tranquility, even if only temporarily. I spent my eighteenth birthday battling with a high fever and an extremely painful bout of tonsillitis. In retrospect, I am sure that being knocked off my feet like this actually did me a lot of good. Away from the pressures of city life and the dance studio, I learnt to shelve of my anxiety. That summer I took a job in Mevagissey, working as a waitress in a quayside restaurant. The following September I moved back to London and took a bed-sitter; first in Chelsea, and later in The Old Brompton Road. I attended a number of auditions and soon secured my first professional work contract and equity card. I rehearsed for a fortnight in Coventry and then danced a four month season at the Alhambra Theatre, in Bradford. Admittedly, the latter engagement took me into the spring of the following year, but even so, I would never be able to squeeze all that into so short a time nowadays!

The show at the Alhambra was quite terrifying in more ways than one. For me, the leap from studio to stage was a gigantic one. In the classroom I had always excelled; I understood what was required of me and felt secure. Here, in my anxiety to please, but also painfully conscious of my inexperience and naivety, I found myself constantly being shouted at for failing to use my initiative. I came to doubt I had any! I had come full circle and was working with Rambert again, in a junior company of graduating students, many of whom I knew from my former days with the school. We worked under the direction of Bridget Kelly, whom I also remembered well….probably for being the most abrasive teacher I had ever met. As choreographer she positively grew horns overnight! Added to my fear of Mrs. Kelly, I found the content of the dancing shallow and meaningless, although undeniably, the training we received was highly beneficial. I felt lonely, miserable and disillusioned. Perhaps, after all, my dreams were totally absurd, quixotic; foolish. I would probably never succeed in this harsh world of theatre and the performing arts. Before the winter of 1965 was through, I had given up chasing the magic of dance.

At last, the season at The Alhambra drew to a close. It hadn't been all bad. In spite of my feelings of inadequacy I had undoubtedly learnt a lot. We had had a white Christmas and plenty of parties, and several of my London friends had visited me whilst I was in Yorkshire. I returned to South Kensington to make up for the six months' training I had missed through illness the previous year. I was sent out to audition for all kinds of wonderful shows but I was still quietly suffering from my nervous disorder. My confidence was severely lacking and Mr. Hardie grew angry with me for my timidity. He was disgusted when I finally signed a contract for a variety show at Westcliff-on-Sea, at the brand new theatre, The Cliffs Pavilion, with the sixties stars Jimmy Edwards, Joan Regan and ventriloquist, Arthur Worsley. The Betty Smith Quintet accompanied us from the orchestra pit.

This time, probably because I had gained a little experience, my choreographer, Bob Marlowe, liked my work a lot. Richard Stone, the producer, also took a fancy to me and gave me a small part in a sketch. It was a court-room scene with Jimmy Edwards as the judge. I was called on as a witness. This was my cue to come mincing on in a bikini, at which point the judge and jury leapt out of their seats and went chasing after me, giving Arthur Worsley, as the criminal, the opportunity to escape. Not the most intellectually stimulating piece of theatre I've ever been involved in! But as time passed, I found that, whatever the show, I was always chosen to act in the sketches.

In 1965, while working at The New Theatre, Cardiff, I had to creep out into the auditorium every evening during the performance and sit, incognito, amongst the viewers. Tommy Trinder then came on stage dressed as a pop star, twanging his guitar and howling into the microphone. My job was to behave like a hysterical fan. I had to shriek loudly, no doubt scaring the people next to me witless, and then stagger down the aisle and make my way onto the stage. I then threw my arms around the surprised Tommy and dropped to the floor in a dead faint, at the same time making quite sure that my bright red, thigh-length, sixties-style bloomers with their black lace trimmings, were suitably revealed to the audience. It was always fun taking part in these ridiculous sketches, and I was invariably presented with signed photographs and boxes of chocolates on the last night.

I remained with Bob for the next three years, following him around the country and dancing in all sorts of theatres; some plush and grand, others smaller and more basic, like the Pier Theatre in Eastbourne, which met an untimely end when it burnt to the ground in the early seventies. I gained a great deal of stage experience, although the work still lacked the depth and dramatic content that I so loved.

Best of all were the ballets. Bob once choreographed a ballet to the theme of a Dégas painting. The curtains opened onto a studio scene, with the dancers in romantic three-quarter length tutus, practising at the barre. The maître de ballet stood in the centre with his stick, and when the music struck up, the scene sprang to life and the 'class' began. What the audience failed to realize was that the 'reflection' of each dancer was actually another dancer working in mirror image to her partner. There was always an audible gasp of surprise when, at the end of the ballet, we split from our reflections and came forward to centre-stage to take up the final scene of Dégas' painting. As I was renowned among my fellow-dancers for being absent-minded, my 'reflection' always gave me a hasty inspection in the wings before we made our entrance. If I had forgotten my black velvet choker, as worn by the ballerinas in the painting, my partner would hurriedly unfasten hers and throw it into a corner, lest the audience should notice the discrepancy and guess the truth!

Another of my favourite parts was that of the drug addict in Bob's modern ballet, 'The Happening'. Provided we worked hard, Bob was an easy-going choreographer. I liked him because he always put me in the front and gave me solo parts.

It was during my second season in show business that I was singled out by the director and handed an important-sounding message. That night the entire company had been all of a flutter. Word had got around that a well-known film producer was in the audience (well known, that is, to everyone except me.

I never could remember such things!) Apparently this celebrated gentleman was much impressed with my dancing and wished to meet me in the bar after the show. I felt mildly pleased, but to my surprise, all the other dancers suddenly expressed a deep concern for my safety. They began warning me of the consequences of associating with this brute of a man who, in their opinion, was only after one thing – and that unmentionable! I didn't think there was much evidence to support this view, but not wanting to be considered forward, I turned him down on three consecutive occasions. I'll never forget the looks of amazement on the faces of the other dancers when they discovered that I had heeded their advice. I often wonder what might have happened had I ventured to use my own judgment.

I sometimes think that if I were to see a video recording of my entire life (heaven forbid!) how much of it would come as a complete surprise. During the years that followed I met so many people, straight, weird or otherwise, and survived such huge numbers of scrapes and adventures, it is difficult to imagine how it all fitted together....or, indeed, whether I remember the half of it. In the sixties it was perfectly usual for me to turn up in some distant location, with all my belongings in a large trunk. This I would leave in the care of the station's left luggage department while I hunted around the unfamiliar town, which was to become my home for the next however-many months, searching for accommodation. It was always good to see Bob next day at rehearsals, and occasionally there was a welcome familiar face amongst the other dancers, but on the whole I was surrounded by complete strangers, many of whom very soon became my greatest friends.

The two week rehearsal period was always extremely tough. On half-pay, we dancers worked, struggled and sweated from morning till late at night as we endeavoured to execute and commit to memory a whole string of new ballets, dance routines, opening numbers, finalés, entrances, exits and costume changes. Almost too tired to eat, we would crawl home at the end of the day and fall into our beds, physically and mentally exhausted, musical scores and dance sequences still throbbing through our brains and eventually spilling over into our dreams.

Between contracts I usually returned to London, where I searched out new digs and a temporary job, either as a waitress or as a portrait or photographic model for the Royal College of Art. (I once received £21 for doing some book covers for three Edna O'Brien novels with Alan Aldridge…a phenomenal amount for a day's work at that time!) Coming home to Cornwall was always a strange but lovely experience. As soon as I stepped off the train…and yes, many of them still puffed steam in those days…it was as if someone had turned the volume button down and put the world into slow motion. I loved it, but work was scarce, and there were no theatres beyond the Tamar. Not even the Theatre Royal then stood across the border in Plymouth.

One of my loveliest memories must have taken place sometime around 1965. I had been living in Earl's Court, waitressing in South Kensington at The Contented Sole, a high-class Edwardian fish restaurant. On the spur of the moment I decided to take time out. I packed my suitcase and caught a straight-through train from Paddington to St. Austell without telling a soul. I had not seen my parents or Cornwall for many months.

Arriving back in my hometown, after a long absence, never ceased to arouse the same sensations. How small and quaint everything looked! The buildings were so clean, the air so fresh, the countryside so deep and green. And myriads of childhood memories popped out to greet me from behind every familiar stone or tree. The friendly Mevagissey bus stood waiting in the station. I boarded it with my luggage, sensing a number of curious glances from my fellow passengers, and settled down in my seat to enjoy the ride home, listening to fragments of conversation in the familiar dialect.

Walking unannounced through the front door of my home, I found my Mum, clad in her customary apron, busy at work in the kitchen. She was so surprised to see me, and I so happy to be home. I had no idea that this was to be one of those unforgettable days, the memory of which would remain with me for the rest of my life.

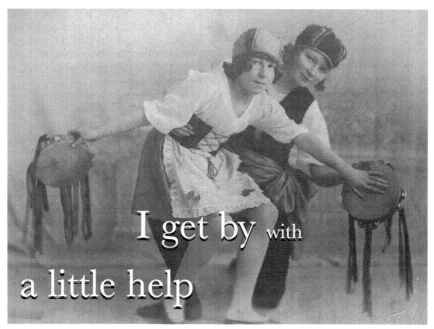

I get by with a little help

from my friends

Elsie and May Enoch in The Tarantella

It was around 1966 that I began 'seeing things' in the night. I would wake up, and finding a figure standing over me, I'd let out a blood-curdling scream. At this point the apparition always disappeared. I don't blame it! Whenever I changed my address I had to remember to warn my landlady about this.

I was terribly naive and used to invent the most dreadful lies in an attempt to dispel the sense of inadequacy which continually plagued me. I took to smoking, in the hope that it would make me appear street-wise and stylish. I was more confused than ever about the incredible beauty of the natural world, music, the arts, and the inescapable fact that the world is such an inanely cruel place, full of injustice and pointless suffering.

I missed the days, and more especially the dark nights, when my Dad and I went for walks together through the country lanes, craning our necks as we looked up into the heavens and tried to pick out the constellations. It was fascinating to feel the benign serenity of those timeless spheres shining impassively down upon us, just as they had spilled their light, throughout the ages, upon countless multitudes of other, long-since departed souls. Unlike my father, with whom I was able to share all my philosophical deliberations and freely discuss the enigmas of life, most of the people whom I met as I travelled about seemed surprisingly shallow. In order to fit in, I decided to live life on two levels: on the one hand displaying a wild exuberance and gaiety, but suppressed beneath this bubbly exterior lurked the unspeakable fear that perhaps nothing would ever make sense, and life was, after all, a meaningless, purposeless phenomenon.

This jolts my memory and transports me, once again, back to my childhood. The year is 1953. I'm standing beside my Mum in Mannings the Greengrocer's, jingling some copper coins in my coat pocket. The shopkeeper, in his brown overalls, smiles amiably down at me and remarks, "I wish I had lots of money, like you, to jingle in my pockets!" I smile dutifully back but inside I'm secretly thinking, "I bet you're not really there at all. You're probably just a picture inside my head." This concept remained with me over the years and grew into a frightening possibility. Perhaps, after all, I was the only real person in the world, and everyone else, and everything I experienced, was just an extension of my imagination. Worse still, maybe I was no more than an extension of someone else's imagination, or even of their dream!...supposing they woke up?

I took to experimenting with marijuana. I had heard this could generate spiritual insight. Nothing much happened, except once, although I suspect on this occasion the substance I inhaled was something other than ordinary cannabis. I found myself alone, and zooming away from Earth in a spaceship. No steering. No hope of return; just limitless, incalculable alternations between barren, lifeless planetary systems, alien constellations and the interminable blackness of empty space. As I shot away, deeper and deeper into the all-engulfing loneliness, the once clear boundaries between space and time became blurred in obscurity. I began to lose my sense of identity. My memory appeared before me in the form of a long internal tube, and losing all control I slipped, and began falling through the inside of it. Far away at the top, people were peering anxiously down at me; a vaguely remembered family with Graham perilously reaching over the edge, arms outstretched towards me. The vision disappeared from view. Desperately, I tried to cling to their memory but it was no use; I just kept falling and falling........ I found myself lying in a deep pit. Other people were there too; mechanical people, robotic, each with a forgotten personal history, working endlessly, pointlessly, at nothing; totally oblivious of each other. A huge, round head appeared out of nowhere: a great grinning god, who laughed mockingly at me and blundered past me into dizzy emptiness.

At last I awoke……. or had I fallen asleep again? It was all the same. I would find myself living in one reality and then wake into another, the previous world having slipped out of my memory like a dream on waking. It happened again and again. Reality was, after all, neither the unfolding of history, nor a stable on-going development of life, but was solely dependent upon whichever dream I happened to be living in at any given time.

With my mind thus engulfed and being drawn, ever deeper, into this confusion of dream worlds, I became conscious of a hand, carefully pulling at coloured threads from pictures of a past life, and weaving them together. A memory was being re-formed. Eventually I awoke once more on Earth, and by incredible good fortune, stayed there long enough to reckon it a constant 'reality' again. I was still terrified of waking up. It took me a very long time to recover from this experience.

✣ ✣ ✣ ✣ ✣ ✣ ✣ ✣ ✣ ✣ ✣ ✣ ✣

The sixties, however, were wonderful! I didn't realize how special those years were until it was all over. I thought perhaps the world always glowed like that for its youth, and maybe it does. Flower power blossomed in our lives, along with love and peace. Men dared to grow sufficient hair to cover their ears and shocked their elders by wearing brightly coloured clothes, sometimes even with medallions or beads dangling about their necks. Oranges and purples clashed vibrantly in every high street; in shop windows, fashion magazines and even on stage sets.

Almost over-night popular music became, not just meaningful, but dripped with altruistic philosophy. Artists like Dylan, Hendrix and Clapton began emerging out of the woodwork in a contagious explosion of creative brilliance. My lonely heart was won over by Sergeant Pepper. The extraordinary lyrics of this unique album captured and epitomized the convictions of the young people of the day. It seemed as if there was a universal desire to do away with pious hypocrisy, and a yearning for the opportunity to embark, each individual, upon a personal pilgrimage in the quest for truth.

Hoards of young people trooped off across India in pursuit of enlightenment, but I was content to do my searching in Clacton-on-Sea. I was *'fixing the hole where the rain gets in and stops my mind from wandering'*(3). But wander it would, across those Elysian Strawberry Fields where I sat alone in my tree(4), surveying, with kaleidoscope-eyes(5), the world as it went hurtling past on its course of futility. All those lonely people.....Where *did* they all belong?(6) In my opinion the song, Eleanor Rigby, is one of the most poignant admissions to the tragedy of the human condition that the world of popular music has ever made.

With the passing of that unforgettable summer of '67, the theatre's winter season loomed once more. I auditioned with a certain Madame Lehmisky, who, it was alleged, expected dancers to pirouette on their eyelashes. I was relieved to find the dear lady considerably less formidable than I had been led to believe. She accepted me on the spot and in early December I packed my bags and set off for Birmingham. It was during this season that I was to meet my future husband.

The Alexandra Theatre, close to Birmingham city centre, is a magical place. In fact, the older the theatre, the more it seems to reverberate with the echoes of performances long past, as if the passions once unleashed upon its stage were so powerful, that they have instilled within the atmosphere a wraith-like aura, which lives on to stir and inspire the hearts of all future performers.

Topping the bill that year was The New Vauderville Band, whose members had recently been enjoying success with their number one hit, Winchester Cathedral. The comedian, Jack Tripp, was also starring in the show. This line-up inevitably called for an elaborate Charleston number. We dancers made our entry for this in a deceptively balletic manner, drifting onto the stage in long, flowing, hooded gowns of a kind of floaty gossamer, but with our fringed Charleston dresses and all the paraphernalia of beads and feathers, underneath. We began with a few bars of a soft classical dance, which was followed by an abrupt change in the music....at which point we flung off our coats and threw them into the wings before breaking into a rip-roaring version of Thoroughly Modern Millie.

Apart from the ballet, a very dramatic affair depicting the struggle between good and evil, and set to music from Gounod's Faust, my favourite dance of all time was the Cancan. Over the years I had become quite extraordinarily flexible, and this raucous dance presented me with the perfect opportunity to revel in unashamed exhibitionism. I just loved the excitement, the energy and exuberance of it all, as we cavorted about the stage in our brightly coloured dresses, shrieking, shaking our flounces and frills, and throwing our legs high into the air. Then, best of all, came that exhilarating leap into the air, landing in jump-splits at the finalé, just as the music reached its climax.

The first half of the show concluded with a very elaborate Scottish Highland scene, when hundreds of gallons of water were used to create gushing water-falls that tumbled down misty mountain pathways, through which the cast descended as we weaved our way onto the stage, making our final entry before the curtain fell. The water was kept in giant containers under the stage, next to our dressing rooms. It must have been an incredibly complex feat of engi-neering to pump all those gallons up through the trap-door every night, cre-ating such an amazingly realistic effect.

Kneeling in the wings each evening, preparing the dry ice for the Highland mist, was a young Greek Cypriot named Dimitri, a backstage worker and the Alex's property master. He had, as he later told me, been 'shipped over' to this coun-try against his will in 1953, when his mother had married an English service man. Dimitri harboured a morbid obsession with death and had a fixation about graveyards. Admittedly, this was pretty grim. However, he also cherished lofty dreams of becoming an artist, or a tramp after the fashion of the poet W. H. Davies.....or possibly even both. This was much more promising!

We first started to converse after he discovered me reading The Philosophy of Neitzche between the matinée and evening shows. I was sitting under the stage in the middle of a huge wicker laundry basket, filled with costumes. I soon discovered that here, at last, was someone with whom I could share my deepest thoughts. Together we would sit, until the early hours of the morning, poring over Thus Spake Zarathustra, the poems of E.E. Cummings, or Dostoyevsky's Crime and Punishment, with The Incredible String Band peel-ing off the Seven Thousand Layers of The Spirits of The Onion in the back-ground. *'You need chaos in your soul to give birth to a dancing star,'* declared Neitzche. True enough! Or alternatively, *'He who blows bubbles shall be exalted'.*(7) (What was he on about?) Well anyway, it was a good enough excuse to go to Woolies and buy a pot of kiddies' bubble mixture to experiment with.

Looking back, I suppose it was really very romantic, as well as quite imprac-tical, that Dimitri should quit the job he so loved, and which offered such good prospects in the area of stage management, solely on my account. But if he had not taken to following me about the country, finding work in whichever theatre I happened to be dancing, I suppose we might easily have drifted apart. The following year we took a bed-sitter together in Eastbourne. I was danc-ing in a show at the Pier Theatre, and Dimitri, after working for a short time in the theatre restaurant, was soon promoted to the position of A.S.M. (assistant stage manager). That year Bob foolishly elected me as head-girl, giving me a position of responsibility over the other dancers. I accepted reluctantly, probably tempted by the resulting increase in my wage packet, small though this was, rather than by any sense of duty or honour. I am afraid I proved to be a very bad one, not having a sufficiently assertive personality to enforce the rules, or to authorize adequate rehearsal practices. I did rather better with regard to the ordering of pointe shoes, making sure I ended up with many more pairs than I needed!

Towards the end of the season I started to feel ill. At first I thought I'd picked up a bug, but in spite of a constant sense of nausea my appetite increased alarmingly! Most of the time I just wanted to sleep, so that dancing became a huge drain on my already deficient energy supply. Particularly demanding was a very acrobatic solo which Bob had choreographed for me. My waistline slowly and mysteriously began to expand! I went for a pregnancy test although I was convinced there must be some other explanation for my unhappy state. On the appointed day I phoned the theatre doctor for my results. Minutes later, feeling slightly stunned but otherwise elated, I stepped out of the phone box and turned to Dimitri. "Will you marry me?" I asked, in response to his questioning glance.

In a whirl of excitement we began making arrangements for our wedding, which we both agreed should take place with as little fuss as possible. The paraphernalia of dressing up and fan-fares had never appealed much to me. Dimitri wrote a long letter home, adding as an after-thought, "P.S. Vivienne and I are getting married on Friday." I phoned my parents, requesting my birth certificate. This immediately aroused suspicion, so I relented and confessed the whole story. They persuaded us to postpone the wedding until the following Monday, in order to give them a chance to make a few hasty preparations, as they fully intended to be with us for the great day. It seemed that our plan for a secret wedding was not to be.

In the end everything turned out for the best. Even the sun shone brightly for us! It was wonderful to be with our families. The theatre cast turned up in force, supplying me with a posy of flowers as well as a wedding cake.

Dimitri and I are the only couple I have ever heard of, before or since, who actually worked on their wedding day. That evening the audience was swelled by the presence of all our wedding guests. After the finalé I was presented, on stage, with an enormous bouquet of flowers and our marriage announced. It was a fitting end to a very special day.

We were to wait another twenty-seven years for our honeymoon, although we did treat ourselves to a trip around London, with a visit to the Tate Gallery the following weekend.

Much to the relief of the wardrobe mistress, who until now had been called upon every week to enlarge my costumes, the show at the Pier Theatre finally drew to a close. Dimitri and I moved down to Cornwall to be with my parents. Demitri junior (Demi) was born the following April, a bouncing eight-pounder with an excellent pair of lungs! I was over the moon!

Motherhood, I understood, was an awesome responsibility, and I was determined to make a good job of it. I was amazed at the psychological changes that took place within me as my maternal instincts blossomed. I remember being astonished, the first time I ever looked at my beautiful son, by the miracle of new life. Not only did he have the correct number of eyes, ears, legs, fingers and toes, but even more incredibly, everything worked as it was supposed to!

I have heard it said that nobody really appreciates life to the full until they have found something, or someone, worth dying for. Life had now afforded me the best possible reason for overcoming the long-term effects of my experience in the underworld, beyond my memory, but this was not so easily achieved. I was well aware that the responsibility of parenthood involved much more than just material provision, but apart from a loving home environment, what else could one possibly offer? Were we all destined to live a totally pointless existence, grow old and die without purpose? If only I knew where to begin searching for answers. Perhaps then I could find something meaningful to offer this trusting little bundle of new life that I had so recently brought into the world.

At the height of the flower-power era I had developed my own kind of joke-philosophy using a hotch-potch of word associations relative to the 'bee', and linked with variations of the verb 'to be'. I had been delighted when, on my wedding day, a huge fat bumble-bee had alighted on my posy of flowers, just as I emerged from the registry office! The general idea was that one should resist the tendency to live in the irreversibility of the past, as well as in the unpredictability of the future, and learn to embrace the present. (Even now I still regard the present as the single moment in time that directly touches eternity). I tried desperately hard to 'bee'....but the sixties were over and it didn't work!

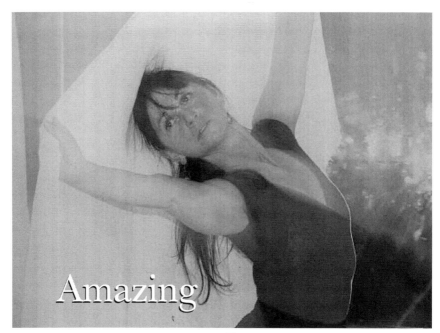

Amazing

Grace

With hindsight, it is so often the chance word, or seemingly insignificant event that influences, or in some cases completely changes, the direction of our lives. There was a day, shortly after my twenty-fourth birthday when, absorbed as I habitually was in my contemplation of the paradoxical coexistence of beauty and needless suffering, I happened to cast my glance upwards to the heavens and sigh to nobody in particular, "If there's anyone up there who can help me understand this enigma, please let me know!"

In retrospect, Somebody was….and Somebody did!

A few days later, in early April 1970, I had a wonderful dream. I came right into touch with the magic! I was walking on a favourite beach of my child-hood. It was deserted, but for one solitary stranger: a man who, to my joy, took me in his arms and began dancing a pas de deux with me. His partnering was perfect, and while the dance grew ever more ecstatic, it seemed as though our very spirits were knit together. In our unity we reached the ultimate state of rapture, so that even gravity had no hold over us. Together we were immersed in the pure essence of the dance!

At last my wonderful partner placed me back on my feet, and without uttering a word, turned and pointed to the horizon above and beyond the cliffs. I gasped in wonder, for there in the sky, glowing with a golden fiery splendour, like clouds caught and transformed by an intense sunset, stood a magnificent church. Afterwards, upon reflection, I realized it did not resemble a typical church building at all, but in that brief moment of time I understood that this glorious phenomenon was, indeed, the true church. I grabbed my baby son's hand (he had somehow turned up as part of the dream) and began running with him across the sand, scrambling over the cliffs in my eagerness to reach that wonderful building in the sky.

Here the dream ended, but I was left with an extraordinary sense of joyful anticipation which remained with me throughout the following day. I shared all this with Dimitri, believing that, if I waited with an open mind, I would eventually receive the interpretation.

Next evening, as Dimitri and I were sitting together in our little home (at that time a caravan by the name of Cara-Van-Gogh) there was a knock on the door. Outside stood a young chap called Mike, a friend of my brother's. Mike was a student at teacher-training college in Exeter, and was home on holiday for the Easter break. We were not particularly well acquainted and he had never visited us before, but I asked him in and it was not long before all three of us became deeply engrossed in a philosophical discussion.

It seemed that Mike was keen to relate to us his account of a remarkable spiritual experience he had had a year earlier. He claimed to have been 'born again' and become a Christian. I had never heard such an expression before. I do not remember exactly what we discussed that evening, but I suppose that, in the case of any such debate, whether one's sympathies lie with a particular world religion, with atheism, or with the insatiable curiosity of A.A. Milne's Elizabeth Ann, the three basic universal questions remain unchanged....
" Who am I? Where have I come from? And what's wrong with the world?"

Until now I had never really taken the idea of a supreme deity seriously, and to my mind, the biblical concept of original sin made little sense. Admittedly, none of us seems to enter life with a clean slate; we are thrust involuntarily into a world that offers no hint of explanation for the purpose of our existence, and we are hopelessly disadvantaged from the outset, inasmuch as our social and cultural inheritance is irreparably marred. It would seem that, just by being alive we are destined to compromise our own ideals and break all the rules! The conscience, while diffusing the light of self awareness into the soul, simultaneously leads us into condemnation, revealing our inadequacies yet failing to offer a solution by which the situation may be rectified.

Socially, too, we appear to be on a slippery slope, being bombarded with conflicting values from all sides. For instance, most of us would agree that it is wrong to queue-barge; the 'I was here first' principle is pretty well universally accepted. This might not cause too much of a problem in the supermarket queue, but where it relates to land, wealth, power, history reveals that it is not uncommon for self-interest to take pre-eminence over the still small voice of conscience. Not only so, but the world tends to applaud such a stance.... *'Steal a little and they put you in jail; steal a lot and they make you king'.*(8)

As our discussion continued, I was beginning to see that an antidote was needed for this condition which the bible calls 'sin'. A rather obsolete word, to be sure, but it did seem quite possibly to be the catalyst that lay at the root of all discord. I learned that this antidote is what the scriptures call 'salvation', and is apparently not attainable through good works, but is an entirely free gift of which mankind is totally unworthy.

The Genesis story, that primitive biblical account of man's origins, is intricately and mysteriously interwoven throughout with a wealth of vital, symbolic, archetypal imagery. Mankind's fatal step in partaking of conscious self-knowledge eventually spiralled downwards into a cataclysmic imbalance of the cosmos, displacing the 'gods' of the ancient world and plunging the entire creation into disharmony. God then provides the perpetrators with coverings of animal skin, thus inaugurating of the rites of sacrificial death; a theme that runs throughout the entire bible, culminating in the passion of Christ, the slain and bloodied lamb of the apocalypse. The phenomenon that we understand as 'the resurrection' reveals how Christ, the substitutionary scapegoat, overcame the ultimate long-term effects of man's devastating fall from grace. And, in response to personal repentance, he is consequently in a position to extend total forgiveness, as well as regeneration, through the gift of his own life.

The debate continued well into the night, and as I pondered these intriguing new concepts, a feeling of excitement began to well up inside me. Until now I had harboured a vague feeling that, if there really were such a person as

God, he would remain outside of the human experience. Nobody had ever proved his existence, and in my opinion, nobody ever would. Could it really be true that God is able to transcend the rationality of our finite minds, and reveal himself to us in some other way than through the intellect? And, more importantly, could the strange events of this evening be, in some way, relevant to the interpretation of my wonderful dream?

Making a pretense at going into the kitchen to prepare some coffee, I left the boys deep in discussion, and crept out into the rambling, overgrown garden, now consumed in darkness. There, in the stillness of the night, I knelt down in the long damp grass and asked this 'Jesus' into my life.

……..All language is generally inadequate to describe any kind of deep spiritual revelation, because words, on the whole, relate only to the physical or emotional realms. Suffice it to say that within a single moment, that illusive magic for which I had been searching as far back as I could remember, was seeping through my entire being, instead of hiding in the shadows, just beyond the next turn in the road. Colours were brighter, and the world was a better place, because I was convinced that somehow, in this complex mixture of beauty and brokenness, there was after all, a divine purpose.

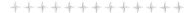

To conclude my story: A few days later, we were introduced to two very interesting ladies: Dr. Queenie Adams, recently retired from her practice in Harley Street, and Ann Whittaker, a medical social worker who had studied at Oxford under C.S. Lewis. Together, these ladies ran a small house-church at Tremore Manor, near Bodmin. After a long discussion, punctuated only by the arrival of cups of tea and fairy cakes, they led an extremely reluctant and sceptical Dimitri into a situation where he was willing to lay down all his intellectual arguments and receive, as I had, this wonderful spiritual rebirth.

As we prepared to make tracks at the end of the evening, I recalled Mike's account of his baptism. I asked Dr. Adams if we, too, could be baptized, and she agreed to make the necessary arrangements. The choice of time and place was left entirely in her hands. I must impress upon my reader that up to this point, I had told no-one, except Dimitri, about my dream. I was as yet very young in my new found faith, and unwilling to volunteer too much information regarding these new, and strangely wonderful experiences. In any case, words seemed quite inadequate to express the way in which the dream had affected me.

One week later, another piece of the jigsaw slotted into place. Our baptism was arranged, and although not quite what I had expected (I had assumed that divine revelation would automatically accompany the experience!) it was not until several months later that I came to understand the full significance of the occasion. For in fact, without my realizing it at the time, our baptism had taken place on the very beach where I had danced with my wonderful dream-partner, just below the cliffs where the vision of the golden church had appeared in the sky!

+ + + + + + + + + + + +

A few weeks prior to this unexpected turn-around in our lives, I had received a phone call from my choreographer, Bob Marlowe, asking if I would consider signing up for another show, which was due to open the following summer. Rehearsals were scheduled to start in May. Dimitri made enquiries regarding accommodation, and we arranged to hire a caravan for the season on a campsite not far from The Ocean Theatre, in Clacton-on-Sea.

And so it happened that just a few days after our baptism Dimitri and I, and thirteen-month-old Demi, trundled off in our little orange mini-van, complete with suitcases, dance gear, cot, playpen and pram, as well as an absolute multitude of other paraphernalia crammed into the back; Dimitri having passed his driving test only the previous week! That night many of our belongings were stolen when our van was broken into.

On the whole it was a disastrous season. Demi objected passionately to this change of lifestyle. He had always been a difficult baby; bright, lively, and quite clearly possessing of a mind of his own. He did not take kindly to being left in the care of his Daddy every evening. We somehow survived the three-week rehearsal period. This is always a tough time, even without the additional

pressures of motherhood. There were three shows to learn, so that the programme could be alternated on a weekly basis throughout the four-month
season. Not long after the opening night I began feeling ill. I soon discovered,
to my secret delight, that I was expecting another baby.

Once the pregnancy was confirmed I really had no alternative but to resign
myself to the fact that my dancing career was at an end. With two small children to look after it would be impracticable for me, and unfair to them, to
continue in theatre work. I longed to leave my job, and desperately wanted to
go home. Demi was miserable. I was feeling queasy all day. It just wasn't going
to work.

The whole unfortunate episode finally drew to a close with my running away.
We stopped off at the theatre on the way out of town to break the news.
Dramatic scenes followed there in the high street with Bob Marlowe, covered
in green and gold greasepaint, waving his arms in dismay as he begged me to
change my mind. I am ashamed to say that I was adamant. No way could I
face dancing until I was three or four months pregnant, as I had when I was
expecting Demi. Away we went, leaving the theatre, and all its magic, behind
us forever…..or so I thought!

✛ ✛ ✛ ✛ ✛ ✛ ✛ ✛ ✛ ✛ ✛ ✛ ✛

The following February our daughter, Emma, was born; another successful
home delivery, and another beautiful, healthy baby. We were thrilled with our
little family, never dreaming that four more babies would be added to it over
the course of the next eleven years.

Shortly before Emma's birth, I had had another very signification dream. I
found myself back in the little cove of my baptism, standing waist deep in the
water. Further out, and much deeper into the water, a man stood, calling to
me in a manner of extreme urgency. He was so intense, almost frantic, whereas I, in contrast, took only a mild interest in his cries.

"How strange," I thought casually to myself. "That man desperately wants to
communicate something which he obviously believes is of vital importance to
me, but by the time his ideas have been transformed into the symbolic form

of words, and those words have entered my hearing, they no longer convey anything meaningful. It's as if he's speaking an entirely foreign language."

At this point, the stranger, who all the while had been drawing closer to the spot where I stood, put his hands into the water and splashed me until my face, head and upper body were dripping wet. As the water poured over me, my understanding was opened, and in a breathtaking instant I heard him speaking the words of life. He had moved further inshore now and stood just a short distance away, across the other side of the cove. Suddenly, I was filled with an overwhelming sense of love for this half-recognized stranger. I made as if to try to reach him, but he conveyed to me, via thoughts, that for the time being at least, this could not be.

When I awoke I knew, without a shadow of doubt, that this was a dream of divine prompting, and the person in the water was that same Jesus with whom I had danced, in the world of my dreams, a year earlier. However, it did seem a little improper that I should fall in love with him! I prayed for whichever he deemed appropriate, interpretation or forgiveness!

The explanation came about three months later, when we were finally sought out by Ann Whittaker and gently coerced into attending a series of Whitsuntide conferences at Tremore Manor. And the theme of the week's teaching? Well, 'The Church, the Bride of Christ'.......of course!

I am sure there are many people have equally wonderful revelations of other aspects of the Godhead, but to me, Christ is the illusive lover of The Song of Songs; the Animus; the personification of the deep mystery of love, whom I have sought after ever since I can remember.

Yesterday Revisited

It's true, it doesn't worry some,
The fact 'tomorrow never comes'.
There's little reason why it should
If all their yesterdays were good.
But if our lives are all regret,
Fears, might-have-beens and unpaid debt,
No soil remains for 'good' to grow.
If only yesterday would go!

If love could rend the bonds of time,
There in eternity we'd find
A perfect garden of delight,
Filled with reason, truth and light.
Our entwined lives would scatter seeds
Whose flowers and fruit would quench all needs.
But death must strike its stinging blow!
Then yesterday … and purpose … go.

Yet love did crush the power of death,
To offer mortals living breath.
There on the cross, despised, in shame,
Love took our anguish, grief and pain.
Futility, creation's cloak,
Subjected so by grace, in hope
That as The Christ in weakness dies,
So shall creation with him rise.
Mercy and truth together meet,
And yesterday falls at his feet.

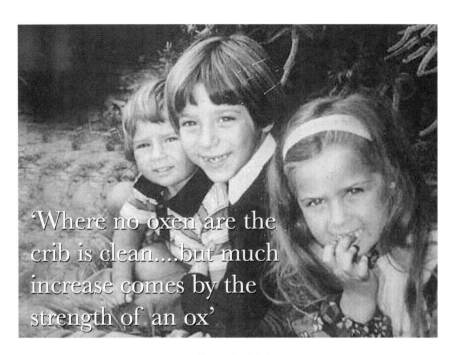

'Where no oxen are the crib is clean....but much increase comes by the strength of an ox'

Proverbs 14:4

Seth, Demi and Emma 1975

Such was my love for family life that, in spite of my aspirations to dance, the desire to have a large family of my own was paramount. I envisaged having four children, close enough in age to play, squabble and grow up together. When Emma was six months old, we were offered a three-bedroom council house in a little village called Bethel, on the outskirts of St. Austell. Situated at the end of a cul-de-sac and adjoining a large, often empty field, it seemed ideal, especially after the confines of the caravan. We soon discovered, how-ever, that many of our new neighbours shared a very different outlook on life than ourselves. Foul language, violent behaviour and theft were common-place. I vowed I would stay for just one year while we looked for something more suitable. In fact, it was not until seventeen years later that we were final-ly able to move away.

In retrospect, it is invariably those sunny carefree days, tinged with the rose-coloured glow of nostalgia, that live on in our memories. Indeed, we did share many happy times during the years that followed. We were fortunate in that we had a fairly large garden, with an apple tree which grew from a mere unidentifiable twig in the first year, to a delightfully tall specimen that waved in the breeze outside our bedroom window. We found that several of our neighbours were good, honest folk, who were no less horrified than ourselves by the undesirable goings-on around us. And best of all, it was while we lived here that four more babies were born into our family.

Seth was the next on the scene, arriving in April 1973. Such a quiet, placid little chap, I could hardly believe my good fortune....until he reached the mobility stage, at which point he was overtaken by a sense of adventure. His brother and sister had both been early walkers, and it was not long before Seth, too, was manifesting a keen-spirited aptitude for bipedal activities. But each time he succeeded in pulling himself up to stand, unaided, on his sturdy little legs, just as the point of take-off, Emma would cry out in an adoring voice, "Oh, you clever little thing!" Whereupon she would rush towards him, throwing her arms around her little brother, thereby knocking him flat on the floor.

With an admirable display of patience, Seth was forced to repeat the exercise all over again, but invariably with the same results. Then one happy day, both older children went together to visit my parents. Left to his own devices, Seth was given the opportunity of a whole day's walking practice, unhindered. He never looked back! His walking and climbing skills developed simultaneously, so that it became necessary to strap him into his cot at night, to prevent him from scaling the bars and dropping out. It seemed that nothing could be kept from his reach. Many a calamity resulted from Seth's indomitable spirit of adventure.

During the summer of 1974 my mother-in-law came to stay, bringing with her an ancient washing machine (the sort with an agitator post in the middle and a mangle attached.) I also had a spin-dryer that danced about the kitchen floor leaving puddles of water behind it. I was thrilled!

The heatwave of 1976 was to set the scene for the next addition to our family. Jude, who arrived that June, made a noisy entrance into the world, crying loudly during the brief interval between the birth of his head and body, but ever afterwards was so contented that I felt compelled to wake him occasionally, just to ensure that he was still breathing. Seth welcomed him into the family with a gift of ladybirds, which he had collected especially for the occasion.

And which I apologetically removed from the little wicker cradle where Jude lay, explaining that the poor insects might get crushed should the baby roll on them.

The excitement of a new baby inevitably attracts the attention of friends and neighbours. Casual callers frequently drop in to view the latest arrival. One of these visitors turned to five-year-old Emma and asked if she was pleased with her new brother. Emma replied that, although she had been hoping for a sister, now that Jude had arrived she wouldn't change him for the world.

Our friend then turned to Seth: "And what about you young man? What did you want, a brother or a sister?" Seth smiled smugly. "I wanted a biscuit," he replied.

As soon as Jude was able to sit up, his greatest pleasure was to spend his waking hours methodically unscrewing all the bolts within reach as he sat in his pram. Remarkably, it never actually fell apart, although I think the hood came off once or twice. I was always careful to fasten everything together before wheeling him from one spot to another.

I sometimes felt concerned that my babies might grow up with appalling superiority complexes, as I used constantly to tell them how beautiful and how precious they were. Thankfully this didn't happen, but it obviously made an impression on Seth.

"Isn't it strange that it should happen to *us*, Mummy?" he mused as he watched me dressing his baby brother one morning.

"What do you mean?" I asked, smiling at the little three-year-old.

"Well, that *we* should be given the best baby in the whole world!"

I have heard many a young Mum confess with a sigh that, after having had two children, the pressures and practicalities of motherhood far outweighed any romantic notions they had previously entertained regarding the joys of having a large family. In my case the opposite happened. Besides, I was secretly hoping that I might eventually even things up by producing a second daughter.

Our fifth child was born just two weeks before Jude's second birthday. My desire for a baby girl immediately flew out of the window. How very glad I am that it was Daniel who turned up that day! I tried hard to spin out those early newborn days, relishing every moment, thinking it unlikely that there would be any more babies to come. Most people seemed to think five children shockingly excessive!

These were such happy times but oh, how busy and exhausting! I always felt defeated by the end of each evening. The daily tasks were insurmountable and many jobs were left untouched, although priorities, like each child's bedtime story, always received due attention. Besides, it was such a joy to re-read and share so many of my favourite children's stories. I'm quite sure my children were regularly deprived of sleep by my eagerness to reach certain highlights in these adventures. I remember pretending to blow my nose, swallowing hard as I endeavoured to relieve myself of the lump in my throat, particularly during the heart-wrenching passages in Heidi, only to find my 'listeners' sleeping soundly, and blissfully unaware of my emotional anguish!

I learnt so much during those early years, especially as we usually lived so perilously close to financial disaster. In fact marriage and parenthood had actually been far more of a learning curve for me than for most of my contemporaries. As I mentioned before, ballet school had little to offer in the area of practical domesticity. The effects of each pregnancy made me so ravenously hungry that I learnt to cook with great enthusiasm, and found the basics of the culinary arts less of a mystery than I had always supposed. I baked bread every day, buns or cakes on alternate days. They disappeared like magic! Orange squash, yoghourt, jams and marmalade, even cheese! Everything was homemade.

I turned my hand to dressmaking. Without any previous instruction I succeeded in turning out numerous children's garments on my ancient treadle sewing machine, as well as making clothes for myself. Externally these creations looked fine, but the atrocities that lay hidden beneath their deceptive exteriors would have given any self-respecting seamstress a heart attack!

I discovered herbal remedies for ailments, and natural foods became our regular diet. My babies might easily have been stamped 'wholemeal and organic' without breaching the trades description laws. Disregarding the advice of my health visitor, I starved (in her eyes) my little ones by denying them anything more substantial than breast milk for the first five or six months of their lives. And although, on the whole, they resisted the much-desired habit of sleeping through the night (could the passage from St. Paul's letter to the Corinthians, *'We shall not all sleep, but we shall all be changed'* really be a direct prophecy to the Tsouris family?) none of them seems to have suffered any lasting damage, in spite of their ill treatment.

55

Regardless of the elements, all babies were transferred to the garden by around 6 a.m. in summertime, or after our morning trek to school (or whenever day dawned) in winter, where they slept (or otherwise) in their prams. Much to my mother-in-law's consternation she once caught me wheeling her grandson out into the garden for his morning snooze, having first cleared the path of snow.

As for as corporal punishment, well, nowadays I'd be locked up! I am ashamed to say that, more than thirty years on, all my fledglings agree that Mum's wooden hairbrush was an instrument of torture to be avoided at all cost. But since at least five of my children turned out to be quite remarkably athletic (possibly a case of cause and effect?) I rarely caught them in the chase. When I did, however, they invariably tried to protect their hinder parts from the neat whack of my flat-sided hairbrush, thus sustaining a sharp rap on the knuckles.

In all honesty I would much prefer to say that I used alternative, more subtle ways of venting my exasperation on my children, but thankfully, they have all grown into reasonably non-violent, admirably dependable adults.

+ + + + + + + + + + + +

One of the disadvantages of having so many children is that, by the time the younger ones come along, one is so busy that much of what happens tends to go straight over the top of one's head. The following anecdotal snippets are just a few incidents that have stayed with me over the years.

Demi, aged six, pleased with his ability to read anything from Ladybird books to the lettering on manhole covers, had developed athlete's foot. I bought a small bottle of brown liquid from the chemist, to be painted in between the toes. At bedtime, when we were due to administer the first application, he emerged from the bathroom looking perplexed.

"Mum, I don't really need to take all my clothes off before we paint my toes, do I?"

"Of course not, dear. Why do you ask?"
"Well, on the bottle it says, 'No dressing is required.'"

As we walked home from town together one afternoon, Demi and I stopped for a while to watch a fat magpie bouncing around the local primary school grounds. Later that evening, when Dimitri arrived home from work, Demi ran up to him and eagerly announced, "Dad, you'll never guess what I saw hopping about in the playground today....a great big pork-pie!"

By the time Emma was able to talk, malapropisms used to roll off her tongue faster than I had time to notice. If Demi had toothache, she would invariably develop 'cornfl-ache'. Always interested in such natural wonders as the life history of the butterfly, Emma once came dashing indoors insisting that she had seen a 'white cabbage' flying about the garden.

From time to time, when the residents of Tremore Manor were away, either on business or on holiday, we were invited to stop over, take a break, and help with the running of the house. On one such occasion, Emma, who had been playing happily in the enormous garden, came scuttling indoors protectively clutching baby Jude, whom she had scooped out of the pram, and announced that a ferocious-looking pig was lurking amongst the bushes. We crept outside, cautiously but valiantly, only to find a large ginger cat standing in the place of the alleged pig. This was not the only time that Emma confused her animal species. She once befriended a bouncy, floppy-jowled dog, but was later unsure whether she had been playing with a bulldozer or a 'boxing-dog'.

Seth was a sweet little boy who melted most people's hearts. He knew exactly how to get the best out of everyone. While his older brother and sister were at school, Seth would amuse himself by quietly getting up to all sorts of mischievous pranks. These included such antics as painting all the mirrors in the house with blue and green oil paint, carefully brushing his curls with the toilet brush before snipping them off with the scissors, then cutting his lip in an attempt at shaving, and finally covering his otherwise naked little body from head to toe in toothpaste.

One morning Dimitiri dropped in unexpectedly from work. As it was nearly lunchtime, I made him a quick bacon sandwich. Seth smiled sweetly at his Daddy and sidled up to him on the window-seat, obviously working out the best approach for a share of the sandwich. Time was short; he needed to work quickly. Then, suddenly...... a brainwave!

"Daddy, Jesus told us, 'Share one with another.'" Good thinking for a three-year-old!

For several years we made regular visits to Tavistock's annual Goosey Fair. It was while I was busily preparing for this outing that I found Seth crying quietly on the stairs.

"Whatever's the matter Sethy-pud?" I asked, giving him a reassuring cuddle.

"I don't want to die yet," he replied sadly.

"What makes you think you're going to die?" I responded, perplexed.

"Well, you said we're all going to heaven today."

Once the difference between Devon and the Celestial City had been explained we were able to go happily on our way.

All too quickly the time came for Seth to start school. Ever popular, it soon became clear that he was endowed with exceptional talent in all sports-related activities. In later years, the school football team, as well as 'Charlestown United', was to become invincible under Seth's captaincy.

From time to time P. C. Stone, the local policeman, was invited to the junior school to talk to the children about issues such as road safety, or the importance of not talking to strangers. Following one of these discussions, five-year-old Seth arrived home from school, obviously deeply impressed; a bundle of papers tucked under one arm, all relating to the topic of 'strangers'. At bedtime he was still talking earnestly of the folly of going with strangers. After a fervent prayer on the subject, he was tucked up and kissed goodnight. I was just about to leave the room when he called me back.

"Mummy, I was just wondering……..What does a stranger actually look like?"

Jude, having developed into a very serious toddler, liked to absorb himself quietly but earnestly in all sorts of exacting projects, such as barricading the front door from top to bottom with a fortress of improvised building materials. His chief passion, however, was drawing and painting. He particularly enjoyed designing greetings cards, and very soon worked out how to make them with moving parts, using pins and staples. Clearly there was another budding artist in the family!

As time passed Daniel, too, began manifesting a marked tendency towards creativity. Music played an especially big part in his life. He also exhibited a gentleness and kindness towards anything living, but in particular towards an elderly blind lady at Tremore, called Daisy. When he was only three years old, Daniel took it upon himself to care for her in an almost obsessive manner, guiding her carefully from one room to another whenever necessary; making sure of her comfort, with cushions for her back and a stool for her feet.

Being dyslexic (although the problem wasn't actually diagnosed for many years) poor Daniel's experience of school was initially very gruelling. He found the supposedly easy things impossibly difficult, and the difficult things easy. He was constantly in trouble for being slow and daydreaming. One particularly bad day during his very first term, he decided he'd had enough. Between lessons he slipped, unobserved, into the cloakroom, put on his coat and started out on the one-and-a-half mile trek home. Thankfully, his teacher noticed his absence and discovered him marching down the school path towards the main gate!

Personally, I have to admire his sense of logic. I remember trying to help him with his English grammar.

"A verb is a 'doing' word." I explained. "It's all about action. Show me the verb in the next sentence in your book." Dan studied the scuffed-up page of his exercise book for a few moments and then announced decisively, "There isn't one!"

Peering over his shoulder I read, 'The dog sleeps on the rug'. "Daniel, can't you see? The verb in that sentence is the word 'sleeps'."

My young son sighed resignedly, as if in recognition of the fact that he would *never* grasp the mysteries of the English language. "How can you call *that* an action word?" he asked scornfully, "If the dog's asleep, he's not doing anything at all!"

As he grew older Daniel's bedroom came to resemble a scientific laboratory, filled with numerous bottles and jars which were connected by plastic tubes, and which fizzed and bubbled alarmingly with all manner of weird concoctions. It seemed quite possible that some day he would inadvertently blow the house up. He was absent-minded to the extent that, while walking the dog through the woods one afternoon, he tied him to a tree whilst he went off to inspect some detail of nature. And there the poor animal remained, forsaken, dejected, and utterly forlorn, until his absence was noticed at dinner that evening!

With hindsight, it is possible to look back on our children's lives and see that, from day one, they each exhibited qualities and characteristics which were markedly indicative of the personalities they would one day develop. Now that he is an adult, with a degree in fine art, we recognize that Daniel is a true renaissance character. He is deeply interested in every aspect of creativity, whether in the many art forms of human expression, or in the natural wonders of the created order and the scientific laws and methods of the great Creator himself.

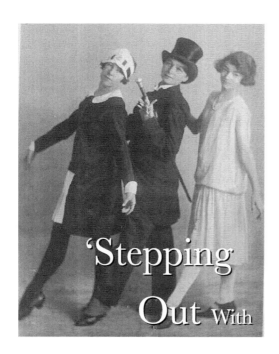

'Stepping Out With

My Baby'

Elsie and May Enoch and pupil

When she was seven years old, Emma expressed a desire to take ballet lessons. This also inspired me to join a weekly class for adults. I felt like the princess in the fairy-tale who came back to life after sleeping for one hundred years, although in my case it was only about ten since I'd been out of the dance scene, and I certainly hadn't had a lot of sleep in all those baby years! It soon occurred to me that there was nobody in the St. Austell area, at that time, who taught modern dance, so I decided to open a class for ladies in the local school. As this proved popular, I progressed to teaching adult ballet, and very soon undertook various classes for children.

Shortly after this development in my life, I received a phone call from St. Austell College, asking if I would act as visiting tutor two mornings a week, teaching both classical ballet and modern dance. The following year, a private school contacted me with an offer of one day's work each week. My life was becoming busier than ever, but how useful we found the extra funds! And besides, dance has such a stimulating effect. I would leave out for my classes feeling exhausted and arrive back home, a couple of hours later, bursting with energy. And just as well – there was still a pile of work to be done!

Somehow I found time to prepare the classes and also to experiment with choreography. I discovered I had so much to communicate! I began planning all kinds of new projects, and in particular a full-scale production called 'Everygirl', using dancers, singers and musicians. We proposed to launch this the following spring. However, it was not to be. To my amazement, I found myself suffering from morning sickness yet again!

It never ceases to amaze me how quickly one accepts, and in my experience at least, thrills to the prospect of a new baby, even if such a thing is far from the planned agenda. And what a very good thing too! It's true we welcomed, loved and enjoyed each child as it came along, but with every addition comes the inevitable increase in the workload. So with all my recent teaching commitments, I couldn't help wondering how on earth I was going to cope.

Lydia arrived in July, 1982. I was, of course, overjoyed. Emma, delighted at having a baby sister at long last, became my right-hand helper. In fact she lightened the workload so much that having six children to look after seemed almost easier than when there were only five.

Indeed Lydia was much loved by all the family. Demi, who from the very outset had adopted the role of the responsible eldest son, was quietly proud of his little sister.......but also took great delight in teasing her! Emma, as I have already mentioned, adopted the role of second mother. Seth, who had previously declared that he couldn't imagine why we needed any more babies, and felt the extra money required to keep one would be far better spent on chocolate, thankfully changed his mind. And both Jude and Daniel, who were now aged six and four years, became adoring, if rather anxiously over-protective little brothers.

Lydia's main problem, and therefore mine, was her tendency to behave nocturnally. As she grew older, far from learning to sleep angelically through the night, she would wake up in the early hours of the morning, usually at around 3 a.m., full of exuberance, wanting to eat, play, sing and party. With a seriously over-crowded household, full of people who needed their sleep in order to cope with work and school the next day, the easiest option was to get up and join in the fun.

I wish it had been possible to capture on video some of the night-time antics of the Tsouris household in those days. The word 'pantomime' immediately springs to mind. Dimitri and I would invariably wake up to find any number of little folk squeezed into our bed in the mornings. Daniel had a habit of sleeping sideways across the bed, so that one of us (usually Dimitri) would end up by being kicked out. He was often to be found next morning, squashed up in one of the children's bunk beds.

I sometimes wondered whether my children resembled me in any way at all. They all looked very Greek, and all manifested passionately volatile Mediterranean-style tempers which were likely to flare up in an instant, causing spectacular scraps and arguments. At least in this way any ill feelings were dealt with immediately. I don't remember anyone sulking or carrying a grudge for more than a couple of minutes. For me, it was much like living on the edge of an erupting volcano. To be fair, I must add that, in public, all the children were so well behaved that no-one ever took me seriously when I complained of being given a hard time. Looking back at this action-packed era of my life, I am often at a loss to know how I coped, especially with the luxury of sleep being in such short supply.

I resisted the 'keep-fit' craze of the eighties on principal for as long as possible, but eventually I, too, jumped on the bandwagon. Consequently I found myself with an additional six hours' teaching for the Adult Education Department. On college days, I would walk into town wheeling the baby in the pram…. either Daniel or Lydia, depending on the year. They would sit, surprisingly cheerfully, watching the progress of the class and enjoying the attention of the students at the end of each session. On Fridays we would dash home, bake a batch of bread and prepare for my three children's classes, which were held nearby in the local school. At four o'clock I would rush off, usually with the long-suffering baby, leaving instructions for helpful little Emma to prepare the dinner.

Holidays away were, on the whole, out of the question, chiefly because it required such a mammoth task of organizational skill to get the family on the road. On several memorable occasions, however, our dear friend Dr. Helen Makowa invited us to stay in her beautiful thatched cottage in the depths of the Wiltshire countryside. Dr. Makowa was a retired lecturer from the London School of Economics; an elderly lady who, at the time of our acquaintance with her, worked for the organization Open Doors, smuggling Bibles into China. It was when she disappeared on these rather hazardous missions to the Chinese church that we were invited to take advantage of her lovely home.

I must admit that dashing about on holiday with a family has always struck me as a somewhat exhausting and superfluous exercise. In any case, we were more fortunate than most, living as we did, in such a beautiful area. Whenever the weather was settled and fine, we would take our large family tent to Pentewan Sands. In retrospect these were such happy, carefree days.

+ + + + + + + + + + + + +

I really cannot write about life with the Tsouris family without mentioning our next-door neighbour, Bill Adams. Bill was a cripple who walked with a stick and carried an enormous chip on his shoulder. His greatest delight in life was winding me up and terrifying the children. To ensure his success in this amusing pastime, he liked to hammer on the adjoining wall of our respective houses well into the early hours of the morning. For his further entertainment, Bill was forever thinking up new and exciting ways of making life as unbearable as possible for our family. These antics included such things as, pretending to run the children over by swerving at them in his car, pointing his air-gun at them from his bedroom window while they played in the garden below, or lighting an enormous bonfire when the wind was in the most convenient direction for ruining my washing. Once, in a fit of temper, he smashed our living-room window with his walking stick.....and then emphatically denied doing so.

Unfortunately for us, Bill's greatest and lifelong friend was P.C. Sandercock, a local policeman. Many a time, after being kept awake half the night by Bill's confounded banging, we would receive visits from this gentleman, with complaints that 'Mr. Adams, of next door, had been disturbed by loud hammering noises coming from our house in the middle of the night.' We were duly cautioned and requested to put an end to our unsociable behaviour!

However, not all the excitement in our lives could be attributed solely to the antics of Bill Adams. We had other colourful neighbours, and one poor chap in particular, who, when he was not resident at one of Her Majesty's penal institutions, would career up and down our road on a motorbike with nerve-shattering sound and speed. He was also the instigator of frequent domestic feuds, evidence of which might sometimes be seen in the form of various items of furniture hurtling out of top storey windows. A few days later peace would be restored, and we all knew that Her Majesty's former inmate had once more been reinstated.

In those days our electricity was supplied through a slot-meter, which frequently ran out at the most inopportune moments. Remonstrations could usually be heard issuing forth from the bathroom, where some unfortunate soul had been plunged, mid-shower, into freezing darkness. Like Sleeping Beauty's palace, the entire household suddenly came to a standstill while one of its members groped around, looking for the appropriate coin, or else went traipsing about the neighbourhood begging for change. This mission accomplished, the next obstacle course was to battle through the side-passage, over bicycles, lawn mowers, garden forks, and other paraphernalia; then clamber on top of the coal bunker and reach for the slot meter. This had thoughtfully been placed as close as possible to the ceiling (sometimes the coin was dropped into the coal at the crucial moment). In the twinkling of an eye light, heat and power retuned, and the place sprang to life once more.

When Demi was seventeen years old, he brought home the most lovable little lurcher puppy named Caz, who completely turned the house upside-down, but very soon became yet another lively and important member of the family. Demi, who was also a great believer in the superiority of natural, free-range products, trained the dog to hunt for rabbits, much to my dismay. He and his friends liked to go 'lamping' after nightfall at weekends, often returning home in the early hours of the morning with the ingredients for next day's dinner.

One Saturday night Demi and his friend Matt came creeping stealthily through the front door at about 2 a.m., both endeavouring to be as quiet as possible lest they should waken anyone. Just as the boys closed the door noiselessly behind them, a shrill blood-curdling scream broke forth from the room opposite, shattering the silence, piercing the stillness of the night and fairly causing the foundations of the house to shudder. Poor Matt, who was totally unaware of my nightmares and nocturnal screaming routine, stood rooted to the spot, quaking in terror and white as a sheet. I don't think he ever dared venture into our house again after dark!

I am sure there are plenty of people who will frown disapprovingly (or despairingly) at my descriptions of life with the Tsouris family. Certainly we come across as a pretty unconventional bunch. But if *'This world is the stunning theatre, workshop, playground of our Father in Heaven'*,(9) it seems likely that the family is the rich training ground for the players, teaching them to appreciate the dramas of the present, as well as preparing them for future roles. How sad it is, in my opinion, that with the current trends of divorce and partner-swapping, so many of today's youngsters are denied the opportunity to be a part of that vibrant, colourful, frustrating, invaluable establishment know as the 'the family'.

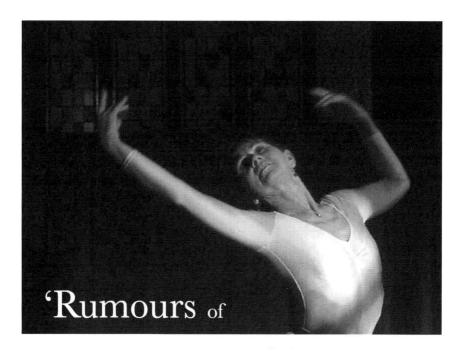

'Rumours of Glory'

I once had a dream in which I went time travelling. During my adventures I stumbled across a couple of tombstones, so ancient that they had long since toppled, and sunk into the ground. As I peered at the semi-eroded inscriptions, trying to decipher the barely legible text of what I had at first imagined to be the names of my ancestors, I was amazed to discover that I had actually shot many hundreds of years into the future, and was in fact, reading the epitaphs of my descendants.

Now I'm going to climb into my time machine once more and travel back to February 1977. At this time we have four children. They are Demi, Emma, Seth and eight-month-old Jude. We have been attending Tremore Fellowship on a regular basis and have found Dr. Adams to be a remarkable teacher, with first hand experience of Middle Eastern culture and customs.

I have been very anxious about Jude for several weeks and am feeling quite worn out with sleepless nights. He has had one chesty cold after another and appears to be suffering from bronchitis. We have decided to bring him to Newquay where tonight, Trevor Deering, a visiting minister, will be speaking and praying for the sick.

I must confess I find these situations difficult. Faith and worry are diametrically opposed and I all too often indulge in the latter, especially when the children are involved. However, when the call for the sick is finally made, I take Jude, who is irritable and squirming uncooperatively in my arms, to the queue at the front of the hall.

I need to stress, at this point, that what I am about to describe actually happened to me in a real and physical way, and not just in my imagination, or as if in a dream or trance. As the minister laid his hands on the sick they began, one by one, to crumple up and sink to the floor. I remember thinking, "Well I hope that doesn't happen to me. I'm holding a baby!" At last Trevor Deering moved towards me. He spoke briefly to me and then, putting one hand on Jude and the other on my head, he began to pray. The room, with its crowds of jostling people, melted away.

……….. I found myself in a beautiful garden, full of June roses and wonderful fragrances. Jesus himself came walking towards me, dressed in a long brown robe. He stood for a few moments, engaging me in the unutterable peace and stillness of his presence, before taking Jude out of my arms and cradling him in his own. I felt the physical release as the baby's weight was transferred into his strong, gentle arms. He spoke to me all the while, in thoughts, telling me not to be anxious. He reminded me that we had dedicated Jude to him as a tiny baby; that he took this matter very seriously and was looking after him. Then he placed Jude back into my arms.

✛ ✛ ✛ ✛ ✛ ✛ ✛ ✛ ✛ ✛ ✛ ✛ ✛

Rather like regaining consciousness after an anaesthetic, I gradually became aware of myself standing in a large hall, with lights overhead and people thronging about me. For a few moments I couldn't remember how I came to be there. All I knew was that something literally out of this world had just happened to me. Feeling slightly dazed, and with a strange sensation in my legs, I made my way to some seats towards the back of the room. My mind felt hazy, but deliciously peaceful, as fragments of my encounter with Jesus began seeping into my conscious memory. Jude, who under normal circumstances would have been fidgeting impatiently and complaining with unrestrained gusto at being kept awake so long after his bedtime, was gurgling happily and catching his breath in excitement.

We travelled home through the night, my spirit seemingly suspended between two worlds as the reality of my recent experience gradually came into focus. I knew that any attempt to put into words what had taken place that night would be futile. In such circumstances human language is wholly inadequate. I had clearly been exposed to a different level of consciousness, and I concluded that, if this was what dying was like, and it seemed it must, then it was going to be truly wonderful!

Jude was still gurgling and smiling blissfully when I laid him in his cot that night. Obviously, something significant had happened to him too. His chest problem very soon cleared up and our nights became peaceful once again. But over and above all else, this profoundly wonderful experience served as something of a lifeline some fifteen years later, when Jude almost died in a horrific accident. But that is another story.

† † † † † † † † † † † †

Up to this point I have said very little about Lydia, except to describe our joy at being given a second daughter, and more importantly, another beautiful, healthy baby. Any frustration I had felt initially, regarding the necessity to shelve my dance plans, very quickly disappeared.

Almost as soon as she could walk, Lydia would join me in my daily barre programme, holding on to the fireguard and hoisting her little legs into the air with an expression of great concentration. She was clearly under the impression that this was all part of normal, everyday life. As she grew older, Lydia's favourite game was 'banks and offices'. She loved interviewing customers, arranging loans, and drawing up financial forecasts. During one general election campaign she even ventured onto the streets with a clipboard, asking passers-by their views on the Green Party. Cheeky, maybe; resourceful, certainly; from the age of about eight, Lydia took it upon herself to write to manufacturers of toiletries, requesting free samples. She was forever receiving exciting little packages through the post, containing fancy soaps, perfume or talcum powder. The companies that she contacted evidently considered her effort and initiative worthy of reward.

In September 1988 we finally made our get-away from the dreaded council estate and moved to Wadebridge, in North Cornwall. During the same month Emma was married. Demi had opted to remain in St. Austell, so for the first time in many years we found ourselves with a reasonable amount of space in the house. In spite of the fact that we lost our home, when it was repossessed five years later, it has been a move we have never regretted.

For several months I managed to keep my children's ballet and creative dance classes running in St. Austell, but this soon proved impractical, the distance being too great for a non-driver like me. In spite of repeated attempts, it was many years before I succeeded in starting any classes in Wadebridge. Following some tutoring which I undertook for North Cornwall Adult Education, I was asked to teach adult ballet to a small group of students at Bodmin College. I had just six very enthusiastic pupils, whose fees did little more than cover the cost of the premises, but at least it gave me the opportunity to rehearse my own work for a couple of hours in a beautiful, purpose-built studio, prior to the class.

I also worked on a voluntary basis at Lydia's primary school, supplying choreography for school plays and teaching creative dance. One day I received a call from the North Cornwall educational coordinator for dance and drama, asking if I would be willing to participate in a huge stage presentation which was planned for the summer of 1992. The project was to involve seven schools and colleges in and around the Wadebrige area, and was to be an ecological musical entitled Ocean World. The story-line centred round a mother whale and her new-born calf, which eventually died in tragic circumstances, due to the destructive and devastating effect of human interference upon the delicate balance of marine life. I was asked to dance the leading role and to choreograph a number of group dances for the children of the Wadebridge Schools. Lydia became my right-hand helper, taking the part of the baby whale.

Several preliminary meetings ensued. I was introduced to all sorts of people who held fearfully important-sounding offices in the education system. On one occasion I was invited to a splendidly sumptuous lunch at County Hall, in Truro, with a gathering of these venerable individuals, in order to demonstrate my choreography and to discuss plans for the forthcoming production. I could hardly believe the respect they showed for my work! Years of serving at the kitchen sink had undermined my self-confidence. The days of my association with celebrated ballet schools and theatrical stars seemed a million miles away. I felt totally inadequate and found the task ahead quite daunting. But the desire to perform had been re-awakened and there was no turning back.

✢ ✢ ✢ ✢ ✢ ✢ ✢ ✢ ✢ ✢ ✢ ✢ ✢

On the evening of December 6th 1991, Dimitri and I were invited to a friend's fortieth birthday party in Launceston. It was a good party, all the more enjoyable since we so rarely went out together in the evenings. We arrived back home at about 11.30 pm. Lydia had gone to stay with Emma for the weekend. Daniel was in bed. Jude was out with friends and had not yet come home. I was rather perturbed by his being out so late, but began making preparations for bed, expecting at any moment to hear the front door bang, heralding his return. Instead, there was a ring of the doorbell, and outside on the step stood the mother of one of Jude's friends, looking frightened and agitated.

Very quickly we learnt the awful truth. There had been a dreadful car accident. Jude and five of his friends had been taken to hospital. All had been released with whiplash and other minor injuries, except Jude, who now lay in intensive care fighting for his life.

The hours and days that followed remain in my memory as a disconnected, horrifying jumble of nightmarish events. As we shot at break-neck speed down to the hospital, twenty-five miles away in Truro, I remember trying to come to terms with the fact that, already, we might be too late. All I could picture in my mind was this trip, fifteen years earlier, to this same hospital, where Jude had been born.

It is not easy to write about Jude's accident. To re-awaken such memories is inevitably a painful process. But all these years later my heart is fairly bursting

71

with gratitude to God for keeping him, and saving him throughout that terrible time. And I am thankful too, for all that the experience has taught me. Jude had sustained severe head injuries in addition to a fractured skull, broken pelvis, cuts and extensive blood loss. When these things happen in films we usually see the family of the injured party anxiously pacing the hospital waiting-room for a few minutes. Then a door opens and a surgeon appears with the words, "He's gonna be alright." Everybody falls about hugging each other and then they go home. Reality isn't like that. No doctor would give us any conclusive assurance that Jude would recover.

For two days and nights I hardly left Jude's side, sleeping upright in a chair beside his bed, watching anxiously as the nurses monitored his condition every hour. As his consciousness began to return, poor Jude became terribly deluded. He spoke in a strange accent, which I found dreadfully disconcerting, and imagined himself in all sorts of unlikely, but terrifying scenarios. There had been a nuclear war. We were in hiding, having survived the initial stages of the carnage. We were characters in a Tolkien novel, lost in the convoluted depths of trickery and sorcery. The hospital ward was a film set. I wasn't Jude's real Mum, I was just acting the part. We were lost on the road that led to death.

One night, about a week after the accident, a middle-aged man was rushed into intensive care with a heart attack. He died shortly afterwards. To shield other patients in the ward from the sense of crisis and emergency, all curtains were drawn around individual beds. Although Jude was incapacitated with his pelvic injury, I had difficulty in restraining him from climbing out of bed as he struggled to "draw back the curtains of death". And in spite of the ongoing state of emergency in the bed opposite, extra nurses were called in to help me hold Jude down and quieten his shouting. Suddenly, after all this frenzied struggling, he lay back on his pillows and announced in a calm, almost robotic voice, "Two angels are appearing on the ceiling."

I have heard of similar cases, where people have witnessed the appearance of angels as they arrive to bear away the soul of a dying person. I believe that, because Jude had, himself, been so very close to death, he was spiritually attuned to the situation around him.

During his long stay in hospital, Jude's friends, teachers and classmates were tremendously supportive. They arrived in droves, or so it seemed, day after day. The stimulation and the memories that they helped to rekindle did Jude a power of good. As soon as his chums arrived he would snap out of the nightmare situations and become almost normal. How I looked forward to these visits! Then, exhausted by the extra exertion he would fall asleep; the friends would disappear, and when he awoke he was back once more in the dark labyrinths of Sauron's treachery, or some similar delusion.

I felt certain that my wonderful encounter with Jesus in the garden, all those years earlier, had been purposely given as a means of sustaining me throughout this difficult period. All over the country, in homes, churches and communities, prayer was being offered up, not only for Jude but for our whole family. When one is left reeling in a state of shock, it is wonderful to feel the support of unanimous prayer. I truly believe that this was a decisive element in Jude's eventual recovery.

I will not tell in detail of the many problems that occurred as a result of the accident. After the initial euphoria of having Jude home with us again, we encountered all sorts of difficulties. He received home therapy for a while, to help him recover the use of the right side of his body. When he was well enough he tried hard to study, but no sooner had he turned the page of his textbook than he had forgotten what he had just read. This led to frustration, which in turn, spiralled into depression. Nine months later he contracted glandular fever.

Early in 1994, two years after the accident, we lost our home. In the end it all happened so quickly, we found ourselves packing our possessions into a rented shed, with no idea where we would be spending the next night. At the last minute, Dimitri spotted an advertisement in the local paper for a small holiday chalet to let. It was situated in a disused airfield about eight miles away. Unfortunately this was too remote an area for either of the two older boys to accompany us. Seth was now working in Bodmin as a sports coach, and Jude had recently taken a part-time job with a silk-screen printer in Wadebridge. The work was not demanding and was proving therapeutic for him. Emma kindly offered to take him in, giving him a room in her converted loft.

That first evening in our new 'home', following the madness of our frantic last-minute move, Daniel and Lydia volunteered to cook the evening meal, using whatever ingredients they could find. As we sat down together to eat, feeling utterly exhausted and surrounded on every hand by the chaos of half-empty boxes, it suddenly dawned on me that, geographically, our family had been split in half. This was a bitter pill to swallow, and seemed far more traumatic at the time than the actual loss of our house.

But more importantly, Jude continued to make good progress, with Emma keeping a watchful eye on him. It was encouraging to see him getting on with life, using his earnings to acquire all sorts of personal belongings: new clothes, books, a TV, his own music collection and CD player. On the day of his final medical check-up with the specialist in Truro, we were aghast to receive a telephone call informing us that, due to an electrical fault, his room had accidentally been gutted by fire. Almost all his clothes and possessions were ruined. As we sifted through the burnt out shell of what had once been Jude's bedroom, we discovered one thing which had remained intact, if somewhat charred around the edges: a scrap book entitled 'My Accident', containing the many Get Well cards and messages from well-wishers, together with a newspaper report about the crash. In a strange way it seemed appropriate, yet at the same time rather pathetic, that this relic, above all others, should have survived the devastation.

Little by little Jude made a complete recovery. In September 1994 he was accepted as a pupil at Falmouth School of Art and was later given a place at Southampton Institute, where he qualified in graphic design. With the compensation money which he later received he sent Dimitri and me to Paris, for our long-awaited honeymoon, twenty-seven years overdue! He bought us a car. Whenever I hear parents complaining about the inconsiderate behaviour of their offspring, I can't help wondering at the generosity that emanates from my own little brood. We are a close-knit family and I am immensely proud of them all.

Jude has become something of an explorer in recent years. He has worked his way around Greece, Cyprus, Ecuador, Mexico, and virtually all the countries of Central America. He has met all kinds of interesting people. He has had his food and water supplies ransacked by raccoons, and then been rescued from hunger and thirst by a coconut that was fortuitously washed up on the Carribean shoreline. He has spent a day and a night lost in the jungle, and awoken next morning to find an anaconda sharing his sleeping quarters. He has shared meals with Indians, scaled mountainous heights and looked deep into the yawning mouths of smoking, ash-spewing volcanoes. As an experienced scuba diver, he frequently explores the fertile waters of the Carribean and the Pacific Ocean, sending home vivid descriptions of strange sea-creatures, and the wondrously exotic fish that inhabit those parts. In Cyprus, on two separate occasions, he was detained by government officials who had decided to press-gang him into joining the Greek army. His surname and appearance apparently aroused suspicion, and he was taken for a deserter. It took no less than a conveniently obliging great-uncle to come to his rescue and vouch for his innocence. In 2002 he embarked on a course at a Spanish language school in Guatemala, and three years later, married Claudia, a beautiful Honduran girl. With his audio and photographic record, as well as innumerable amusing, often hair-raising anecdotes, he could easily write a book of his own and will probably do so in the course of time.

It might seem that I have deviated a long way from the preparations for Ocean World, but in fact the story of Jude's accident turned out to be most relevant to this work. Once the rehearsal period was over and the show, which ran for three nights, was staged, it drew crowds form all over North Cornwall. The huge auditorium was at bursting point and still people were being turned away. The production was an enormous success. Overnight we all discovered how talented Lydia was. It had never occurred to me that she would be anything other than perfect for the part, but then again, neither had it occurred to me that my expectations might be too high. Whatever the case, she intuitively imbibed the ethos of the story and became the embodiment of new birth, playfulness, vulnerability and pathos as the drama unfolded.

To my wonder, I discovered that my own involvement with the role of the mother whale became an important part of the healing process, following the trauma of Jude's accident. As I danced the final scene, expressing my grief at the loss of my baby, all I could see in my mind's eye was Jude's bloodstained, distorted face as he lay, unconscious, on the hospital bed, surrounded by pools of blood, and with myriads of wires and tubes attached to his body. What a powerful medium dance can be when it comes to unloading our emotional baggage. Little wonder there wasn't a dry eye in the house! This was a turning point for me. I felt I had truly become a dancer again. I had received recognition in my own town. It felt so good! Even now, all these years later, people in Wadebridge still remember Ocean World.

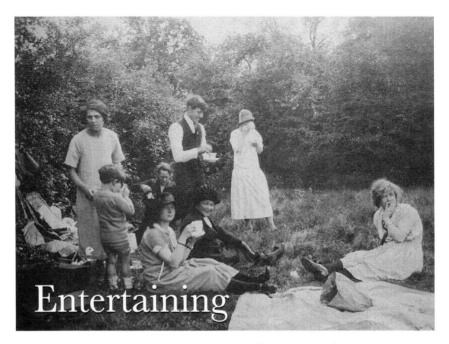

Entertaining

Angels

Family picnic at Hilly Fields, Enfield, early 1920's.
May and Emily Enoch seated centre

'Life is just like a merry-go-round, with all the fun of the fair.....' So goes the song. Well maybe, but after a bad experience inside a blacked-out house with collapsible floors and ceilings at a fun-fair in the sixties, I prefer to compare it to a children's playground; the various apparatus providing a sufficiently hazardous appeal, yet within a reasonably safe environment.

I remember, as a very small child, braving the swings and roundabouts in the park behind my Grandma's house. I even occasionally took my chance on the witch's hat. But that huge, sky-scraping monstrosity, the slide...well, that was something else! I recall watching, with great admiration, all the other brave souls who scaled with nonchalant ease the dizzy heights that topped those daunting metal steps. How grand it must be to sit poised at such an altitude one moment, and then go plummeting back to earth with the wind rushing through one's hair the next! On more than one occasion I actually mustered sufficient courage to climb the steps, taking my place in the queue with the other children…only to lose my nerve once I reached the top. Then followed the humiliating descent….not in the right direction, I hasten to add, but backwards, down the ladder, treading on the toes of all those other intrepid youngsters, who stood clutching the hand-rail, pulling in their tummies in order to let me squeeze past.

If life can be compared to taking one's turn on the slide, the ascent must represent the years from birth to adulthood. This seems to take forever! Then follows a lengthy interim period when one hovers on the top rung. From this vantage point it is possible to look back on one's childhood, as well as way into the future, where old age and even mid-life appear to be still far, far away in the distance.

I've never been quite sure what is supposed to happen next, but in my case I suspect I was pushed. Either that or I slipped. But then again, perhaps it is all just a natural progression. Suddenly I find myself hurtling through the stratosphere of time at a previously unimaginable rate. I still have so many tasks to complete, such a huge array of unfinished projects, I just hope I don't reach the bottom too quickly!

One's memory, however, is such a wonderful asset. Through its miraculous powers one is able to retain a lifetime of experiences, significant or otherwise, which occur either during the slow upward climb, the interval at the summit, or as one makes one's swift nosedive towards base. And it is to be hoped that these same memories serve to season one's life with a little wisdom. Certainly some of the following anecdotes make me cringe when I think of the things we used to get up to!

✦ ✦ ✦ ✦ ✦ ✦ ✦ ✦ ✦ ✦ ✦ ✦ ✦

Although, as our family grew larger, our home seemed to shrink correspondingly, yet from the very outset we adopted a policy of hospitality, particularly towards down-and-outs. Our first customer was a fellow called Phil, who took over the living-room of our council house for a couple of months while sorting his life out. I remember very little about him, other than he seemed to have no family to support him. At this particular time he just needed a little extra encouragement and friendship. He arrived accompanied by a somewhat unpleasant odour, which improved considerably, along with his general appearance, during the weeks he spent with us. The last we heard of him was that he had found a job, married and settled down quite happily.

Ruth was a girl of about nineteen who lived with us in St. Austell for a much longer period of time. She actually paid a contribution to food costs and was quite helpful with the children. Ruth was beset by many problems, however. In the end I fell out with her over a number of stories she had spun about us and our friends. Looking back, I think I managed the whole episode very badly; it was certainly a learning period for me. I deeply regret having lost contact with her as she was a lovely girl in many respects.

Early in 1980 we took our family, along with our latest guest (a girl who had suffered considerable abuse at the hands of her father, as well as from connections with the occult) to visit a rehabilitation centre near Clapham Common. Dr. Adams and Ann Whittaker were trustees of several of these homes, which had been set up during the late sixties in order to help ex-drug addicts and prison offenders. Here we met Danny, a child-like, gentle giant in his late twenties. He took to us all with great enthusiasm. Later that year his house-parents consented to his coming to stay with us for a week or two. As we had never been fortunate enough to possess a spare bedroom, this meant accommodating him on our new settee; our most respectable item of furniture, bought at a real bargain price at a local sale.

Towards the end of his holiday, Danny appeared to undergo a change of character. He bitterly resented the fact that he had to return to London. On his last night, in an act of defiance, he insisted on consuming several cups of coffee after 6 p.m. (we had been warned not to let this happen.) The result was that, after his departure, I found the seats of the settee soaked with urine, and then turned over in the hope that we wouldn't notice. The covers were not removable, so could not be washed. Our prize piece of furniture was good for nothing but the rubbish tip!

I learnt a lot about time-wasters during those years; people who enjoy nothing better that to soak up the sympathy, energy and time of anyone soft or silly enough to listen to them. I was all of that to begin with, but have learnt to be more discerning and a great deal harder in recent times.

Of course, not all our 'angels' stayed for long periods of time. There were a lot of one-nighters, most of whom I have since forgotten about. Ken Jenkins and his aged dog were probably the only senior citizens who spent their holi-day breaks with us. It was quite amazing how many vagabonds and ex-pris-oners we attracted! One fellow came knocking on our door at around mid-night one dark night, asking if we would give him a lift to a neighbouring vil-lage. Dimitri promised to take him in the morning if he agreed to sleep on the settee. It later transpired that our guest had been discharged from prison only that morning, and was a recent convert to Christianity. We, presumably, were the answer to his prayers!

Whether of late I have suffered a decline in compassion, or an increase in wis-dom, is debatable. I have to admit, I would be far more reluctant to allow any suspicious-looking character into my home these days, especially if there were young children about. It is true to say, however, that whenever strangers were abroad in our house, I rarely had more than a wink of sleep.

After moving to North Cornwall, it was invariably our own teenagers who turned up with the waifs and strays. At that time we held regular 'family coun-cils', when the whole clan met together to discuss anything from their individ-ual grievances, to school concerns, to their views on popular music. Social jus-tice also featured high on the agenda.

One evening Jude rang us, requesting that we take in four stranded young men for the night. These bedraggled individuals had wandered in to the Sunday evening church service with a sad tale of a broken down vehicle, very little money and nowhere to stay. Obviously they were hoping for a soft touch. Not surprisingly, everyone with a spare bedroom was otherwise engaged that night. Jude immediately volunteered our hospitality.

The four arrived in a cheery state, demolished huge quantities of tea and toast and helped enthusiastically with the sorting of blankets and pillows while we arranged makeshift beds all over the living-room floor. We sat up into the early hours, discussing life, the arts, philosophy. I related the story of my conversion, and this really seemed to interest them. We all had a great time together.

Next morning some of the more mechanically-minded church members got together and helped to fix the troublesome vehicle. By lunch-time our new friends, and their van, were ready for the road. A few days later, we learnt that all four of these nice young men were on the run from the police, and had been arrested shortly after leaving the county.

Several months after this episode, I received a letter from one of them, thank-ing us for our hospitality. Warren, as our friend was called, was currently serving eight years in Exeter prison for armed robbery. He had become a Christian and was bubbling over with his new-found faith. I continued to correspond with Warren for some time, sending him tapes and other small gifts. Eventually he was moved to another prison and we lost contact.

As I write, memories of other colourful characters come flooding back. Isa was a gregarious, larger than life Brazilian woman. We had met when she stopped me in the street, asking me in her broken English where she could get her shoes mended. She chattered on in a friendly manner, and thinking she might be feeling lonely in a foreign country, I foolishly gave her my phone number. From that day on, Isa constantly invaded my time and privacy, turning up at the most inappropriate moments, usually when I was in the middle of cooking dinner. She would come bursting into the kitchen, shrieking in anguish, describing how she had just escaped death at the hands of her fiancé. With graphic descriptions, and a dramatic display of play-acting, she would demonstrate how her lover had attempted to cut her throat while she clung to him in a passionate embrace.

One night I agreed to accompany her on a search of all the local pubs in order to help find the fugitive, who had apparently gone missing after their latest brawl. We eventually discovered him sitting in The Swan, eating cod and chips. Isa rushed up to him announcing, "Ah, Massimo! Here is Vivienne. She is come to tell us about the angels!" I did my best to keep a casual distance from her after a few more of these episodes. Nevertheless, Dimitri and I ended up attending their wedding and later writing to Massimo while he was in jail.

The very fondest memory I have of any of these angelic visitors is of a sunny-faced, curly-headed boy of about twenty, named Dale. We were on our way to visit friends in Mylor Bridge one day, when we saw him alternately juggling and hitching by the roadside. We picked him up and chatted all the way to Falmouth, where he left us. I forget where he had come from, but he was spending that whole summer travelling about the country, looking at life. We gave him our address, should he need a place to stay overnight on his return journey. A couple of weeks later Dale rang us. He had decided to take us up on our offer.

There was nothing particularly remarkable about his stay with us, except that he proved to be one of the loveliest, most thoughtful, unpretentious people I have ever met. He loved the children and tried with great patience to teach Daniel and Lydia to juggle. He later told us that, while he had spoken of his wanderings in a geographical sense, it was really a spiritual journey he was seeking. He asked a lot about our beliefs and one morning confessed to hav-

ing 'said the words', but was not sure at that stage whether anything significant had happened. We did our best to reassure him and he left us soon afterwards to continue on his travels. We will always remember Dale with great
affection. I hope with all my heart that he has found what he was searching
for on his pilgrimage.

+ + + + + + + + + + + + +

In 1989, Emma and her husband Pete turned us into grandparents, with a
repeat performance fourteen months later. From the outset it had been bla-
tantly obvious to everyone, except Emma, that this marriage was destined to
end in disaster. Pete, initially a pleasant enough person who positively oozed
natural charm, was the product of a broken home, unstable in all his ways.
Work was not something he was accustomed to, except for occasional, casual
spurts, which always ended in the proceeds being blown away on alcohol.
There developed an endless cycle of splitting up, affairs, forgiveness and reconciliation.

Just before Christmas 1992, during an unusually long separation, we succeeded in finding Emma a house to rent, just a few doors away from our own. The
following January, her third child, Jasmine, was born. The new home presented too good an opportunity for Pete to miss out on. In fact he did, at that time,
seem genuinely fond of the children, although it never occurred to him that
he should bear the responsibility of providing for them. He soon moved in to
be with his family and so the cycle continued.

One very wet August afternoon of that same year, Emma called in to see me
on her way back from town. Apparently, while she was out shopping, a man
had approached her, seeking her advice. It seemed that he and his nephew
had been walking the coastal paths for several days and they, as well as all their
belongings, had become soaked through with the incessant rain. He asked
Emma whether she, or anyone she knew, would be willing to help them.
Feeling that this was a little strange, Emma told the pair to wait where they
were, and then came rushing to me for advice. We decided to invite them back
for a hot drink and take it from there.

Before long the young man, whose name was Anthony, and his twelve-year-old nephew, Laslo, were sipping tea in the living-room while their clothes and sleeping bags steamed over the radiators. I soon decided there was nothing too alarming about them and so offered to put them up for the night. (It actually turned out to be a week, but I'm not sure where they slept!) Over dinner that evening Anthony looked at me questioningly. "Why are you doing this?" he asked. "Not many people would open their homes to complete strangers."

"Well," I replied, "There's a verse in the bible that tells us, *'Show hospitality towards strangers, for in doing so some have entertained angels unawares.'*(10) For all I know, you two might be God's messengers in disguise!"

At that point Anthony's jaw dropped open. "I'm certainly not an angel," he replied, "but I *am* a Christian! I work with The Jesus Army in London, helping street people." All of a sudden there seemed to be an awful lot to talk about!

The following day Anthony asked me, "Is there anything I can do for you, in return for having us stay here?"

"Not really," I responded, "although there is one thing. You can go across the road and visit my daughter if you like, and help her to rediscover her faith."

And that's exactly what happened. It was a long, hard, desert experience for Emma during her eight years of marriage to Pete. Then there followed the inevitable divorce, and all the difficulties of having to cope single-handed with her emotionally confused little family. This eventually culminated in a complete nervous breakdown; a very frightening time for us all.

In October 2001 we were overjoyed to see her happily married to Chris, a responsible, hard-working, dependable fellow, whom we all love dearly. And who, as I like to remind them both, is a complete answer to our prayers. If for no other reason than Emma's return to faith, I guess I'm glad we were foolish, and naïve enough, to open our home to so many of those strange angelic beings.

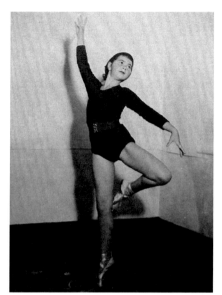

At twelve years

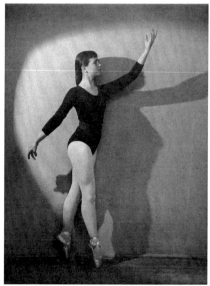

At thirteen

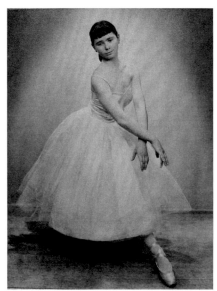

On my acceptance by The Rambert
Ballet School, London in 1959

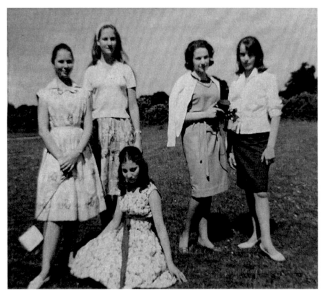

With friends in the grounds of Tring Park.
Left to right: myself, Harriet Oakley, Valerie Hilditch,
Jeanette Nathan, Helena Szchaulska

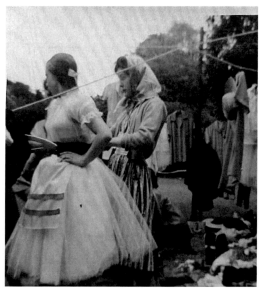

*Rehearsals for Parents Day 1961,
The Elizabethan Gardens, Tring Park*

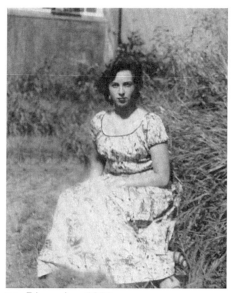

Diana circa 1955

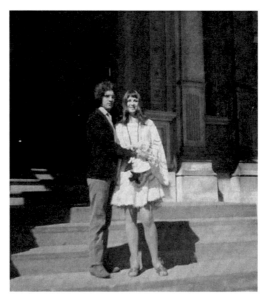

Dimitri and me on our wedding day 1968

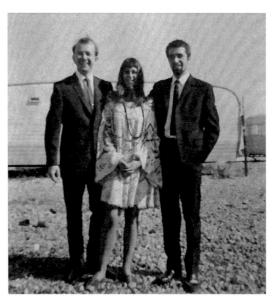

Barrie, myself, Graham

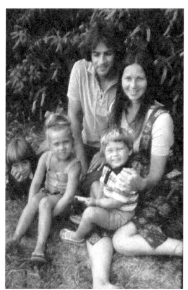

*Dimitri and myself with Demi,
Emma and Seth in 1975*

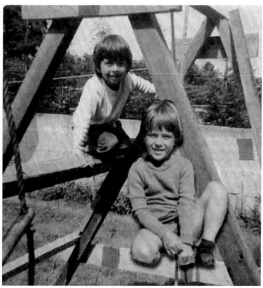

Daniel and Jude in 1982

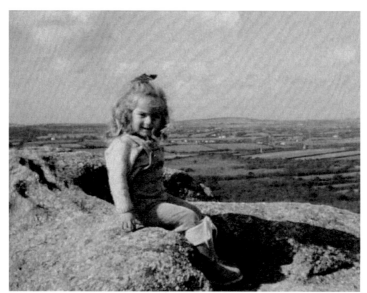

Lydia at Helman Tor in 1985

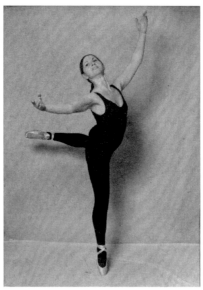

Rehearsing for Everygirl in 1981

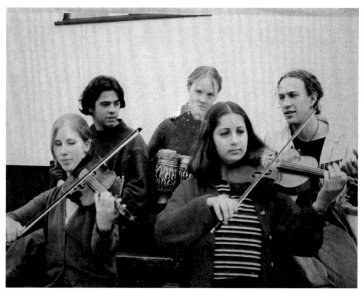

The Elastic Band in 1996. Left to right: Jennie Sanderson, Daniel Tsouris, Meg Lamond, Lydia Tsouris, Joe Webster.

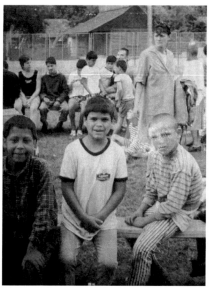

Orphans at Remitz Orphanage, Romania

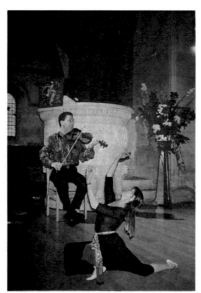

*Dancing with Paul Heyman in
Cambridge, 1999*

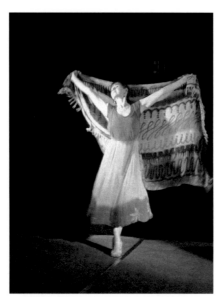

*Dancing 'The Lament of Jephthah's
Daughter' in Thessalonika, Greece, 2003*

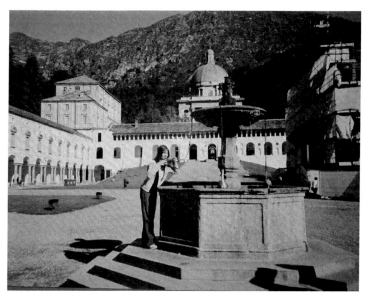

The monastry at Oropa, Northern Italy, 2002

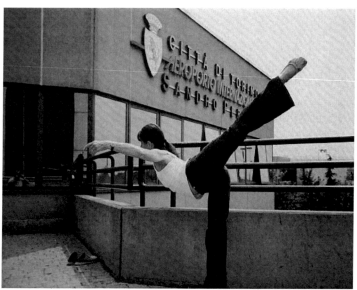

Practising in Tourin airport after missing our flight

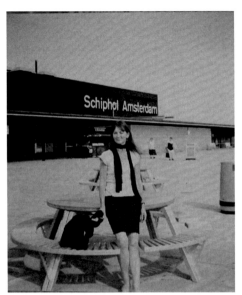

At Shiphol airport, Amsterdam, 2003

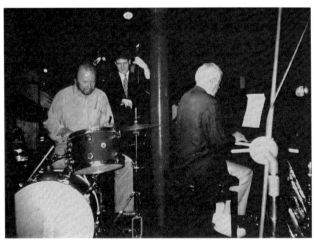

Barrie, (drums), who went on to play in various TV and radio shows, as well as with a number of well-known bands, nationally and internationally. He has accompanied such celebrities as Humphrey Littleton, Alex Welsh, and Fred Hunt. He has had the honour of playing and recording alongside many of America's legendary jazz heroes, including Billy Butterfield, Bud Freeman, Buddie Tate, Wild Bill Davidson, Eddie Miller, Ralph Sutton, and Dick Wellstood.

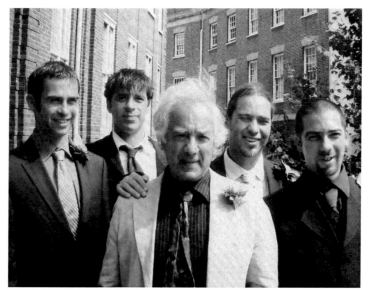

Left to right: Daniel, Demi, Dimitri, Jude and Seth at Daniel's wedding in 2008

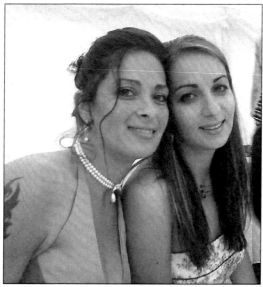

Lydia and Emma in 2007

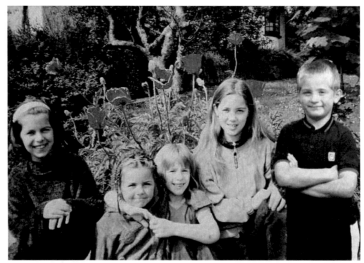

Grandchildren Katie, Jasmine, Jessica, Natalia and Danny in 1998

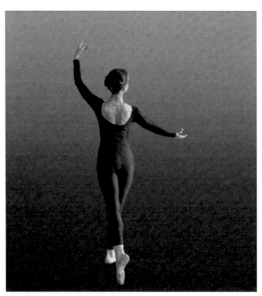

Rehearsing in 2008

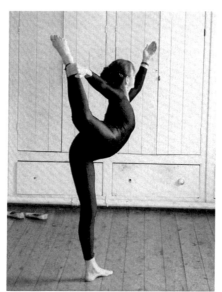

The final curtain. Myself at 62.

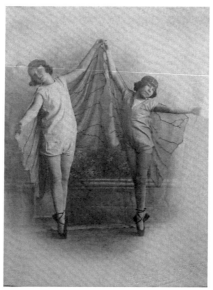

May and Elsie in 'Butterflies' circa 1919

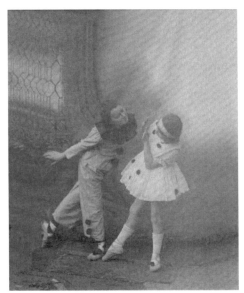

May and Elsie in Le Carnaval circa 1920

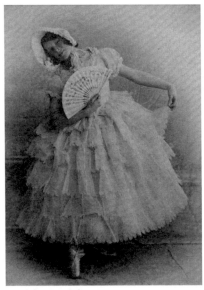

May aged fourteen years

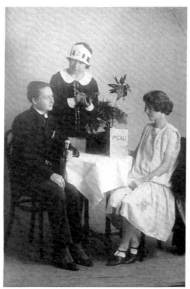

Above, dance sponsored by Lyons Corner House. Below and overleaf, the local children of Enfield who attended May's free dance sessions. Concerts arranged and choreographed by May, aged fourteen. (Note the elaborate costumes!)

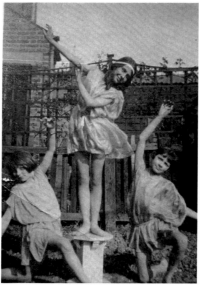

Greek dancers

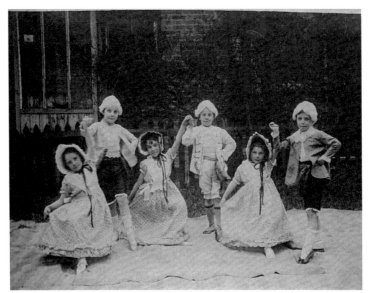

Minuet

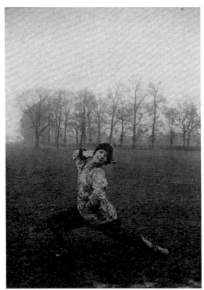

May in her Russian costume

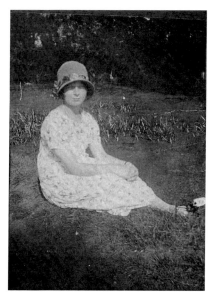

May circa 1927

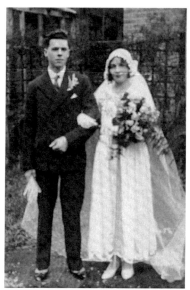

My parents' wedding in 1930

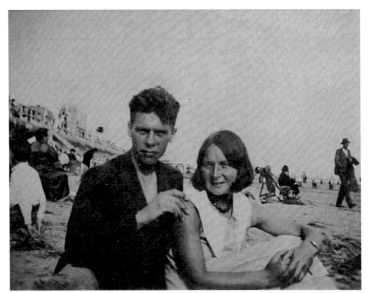

My parents – a day at the seaside

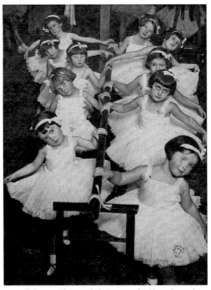

Diana (front right) at a ballet class in 1934

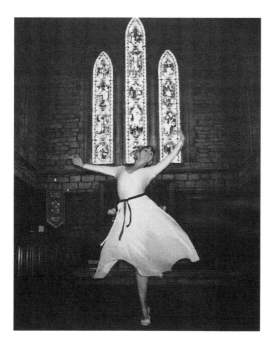

'Better To Light a Candle than Curse the Darkness'

All that I have described so far, in relation to family life, demonstrates the value of interdependence, the importance of 'give and take', and the recognition that, while each of us is far from perfect, we all have value. Let's face it, we need each other, and good relationships don't just happen. They require determination and perseverance as we come to terms with the faults and inconsistencies within the personalities of our loved ones, and more especially, within ourselves.

Paradoxically, a touch of what some might term 'self-sacrifice' invariably leads to self-fulfilment. On a personal level, although I forfeited my dance career in favour of raising a family, it is because of my experiences of motherhood that my creativity has developed far beyond my wildest dreams. Indeed, I have so much to be thankful for which, were it not for my children, I would never have had the opportunity to be involved in. A good example of this has been our association with The White Cross Mission.

In addition to her acting and dancing achievements, Lydia also showed considerable musical talent. This led to a very busy lifestyle. She soon found herself playing flute in the church music group, and violin in two local orchestras. Then, at the age of thirteen, she was invited to join a folk group called The Elastic Band. The group members were planning to raise enough money to take themselves, and their music, out to Romania to work with orphaned children.

We very soon discovered that Daniel, who was quietly developing into a dedicated young artist, had similar musical aspirations. The chief difference being that, whereas Lydia constantly aired her desire to play just about every musical instrument under the sun, Daniel, with his unobtrusive disposition, failed to alert our attention to his wishes for the same. To compensate, we bought a guitar for his sixteenth birthday and arranged a course of private tuition. Whenever he was not painting or sculpting, Daniel was studiously practising his music. Within a remarkably short space of time he, too, became an accomplished member of The Elastic Band.

The Elastic Band, so named because of its tendency to expand and contract according to the number of young people involved in it at any one time, was a folk group that played mainly Irish and English reels and jigs, with a variety of Levellers songs thrown in. There were numerous rehearsals, often held in our house. Dimitri helped with booking arrangements and generally acted as a kind of roadie for the group. Throughout the busy summer months they played several nights a week around the pubs of North Cornwall, raising money for The White Cross Mission, a Truro-based organization that helps with the running of two Romanian orphanages, as well as buying and establishing homes for smaller groups of children, and training local carers to act as house-parents.

For three consecutive years The Elastic Band took their music to the orphans of Romania. Emma also travelled out with them as an aid worker. Dimitri and I followed in the summer of 1996. This trip proved to be the experience of a lifetime.

The White Cross Mission is a charitable organization set up by the Rev. Pat Robson in the wake of the collapse of the Ceausescu régime, and in response to the shocking discovery of hundreds of traumatized children living in appalling conditions, many of them never having seen the light of day. I tried hard to prepare myself for my first encounter with the orphans, knowing it would be a harrowing experience. In spite of my efforts to steel my emotions, I remained in a state of shock throughout the first day.

In this kind of establishment there are almost as many tragic stories as there are children. We came across cases where children had been blinded by being repeatedly beaten about the head. Almost everyone had ugly scars on their bodies. It was impossible to tell who was mentally unstable and who was simply traumatized. Until The White Cross had intervened it had been customary to tie babies and small children to their cots all day, in order to minimize the work of their 'carers'. This resulted in impeded development in such areas as coordination, speech, and the ability to relate socially, as well as in stunted growth. There were those to whom daylight was abhorrent, presumably because they had become accustomed to living in darkness. Or perhaps they found the prospect of the outside world too frightening to face up to. Whatever the reason, these children kept themselves hidden away, concealed under blankets, isolated, silent, uncommunicative.

Apart from these pitiful cases, a few others remained detached, distancing themselves from the crowds and the general excitement that occurred whenever an outsider entered the orphanage gates. Most, however, were overwhelmingly friendly and treated us like human climbing frames. All the orphans looked like little boys, their hair having been closely cropped in order to avoid the problem of head-lice. Anyone with long hair, like mine, was an object of fascination to them. On my very first day in the orphanage I was taken to Salon Six, where many of the worst cases were currently receiving therapy. The moment I entered the room, three children leapt at me. The smallest climbed into my arms and clung to me, sobbing, a second grabbed my legs, almost knocking me over, while a third swung from my hair. By the time I had fought my way free I was shaking from head to foot and had lost a good deal of hair.

Camping in a deep valley at the foot of the Transylvanian mountains, amid stunning scenery and surrounded by the peasant farming community, proved to be a unique experience which will remain with us forever. This was not a time for enjoyment, as in the sense of a pleasurable holiday, but had a far more significant and lasting effect upon us. To witness the trauma of these beautiful children, but also seeing the extent of human goodness in those who reached out to them, was a truly humbling experience.

Also travelling and working with us was Sacred Turf, another Cornish-based folk-rock band. This was an older, more experienced group of semi-professional musicians, who had previously put a great deal of effort into the fund-raising schemes. After our day's work in the orphanages, both bands played together in the local taverns for the peasants and villagers. This was very well received by the whole community, as well as being great fun for all of us. The free entertainment proved invaluable in helping to bridge the divide between the villagers and the orphans who, being mainly of gypsy origin, were great-ly despised by the majority of 'respectable' people.

One hot sunny day, the administrators of the orphanage granted us a free afternoon, giving us the opportunity to attempt a little mountain climbing. We set off in high spirits, a party of about twenty, following the mountain path, which became increasingly precarious the higher we climbed. I am always fas-cinated by unusual flora, and after lingering in the lanes to examine the beau-tiful mountain flowers, I was a little perturbed to find myself alone. Dimitri and the others had evidently gone striding on ahead. It was tough going, but the adrenaline generated by my anxiety served me well. A couple of hours later, after a long and strenuous climb, I arrived at the top, red in the face, limbs shaking, only to find that I had out-stripped Dimitri, who was still far away on the lower slopes. All the young people expressed their admiration at my apparent fitness. Little did they know the true reason for my swift ascent!

The following year, Emma and Lydia really did find themselves separated from the main party while climbing this same mountain. As night closed in on them, they were horrified to hear the baying of wolves getting ever closer! Stories of Count Dracular and his band of Transylvanian vampires did little to assuage their fears. Although the wolves continued to follow them from a distance, the two girls eventually succeeded in finding their way back to the camp, both vowing to be more careful in future!

At last our time in Romania drew to a close. On the return journey, as on the outward trip, we spent a night in Budapest and another in a little village close to the French-German border, where our accommodation was taken care of by a generous church community. In all it had been a bitter-sweet experience. As an individual I felt I contributed very little. As a group I believe we brought a great deal of joy and colour into the somewhat grey world of a good many children.

Eventually The Elastic Band disbanded (a fitting way to describe the dissolu-tion of a music group!) due to the five remaining members (it had shrunk!) leaving the area for their various university locations, or other places of employment. We remain in touch with Pat Robson and continue to fund raise for the cause. Perhaps one day we will return. Who knows?

Song for Romania

We're glad you've come to visit us,
It's good to know you care,
You friends from distant England,
With your gifts and love to share.
The magic that you bring us,
Of colour, dance and song,
Stirs deep within this clouded heart;
Makes me wish to belong.

Look into my dark eyes
And there you may find
A fearful, haunted passage-way
Into my troubled mind.
Fear, rejection, helplessness,
Each has left its mark,
Like fleeting ghosts of memories
That dance there in the dark.

Remember us when you return
To your world, so rich with choices.
Our prayers are whispered on the air
Though the wind may drown our voices.
Will you speak for those who have no voice?
Will you act for those rejected?
Would you help to heal one anguished heart
And shield the unprotected?

Some day you'll find someone to love;
Yes, I really hope you do.
I dare not hope that I might find
Someone to love me too.
When you stand there by the altar,
In your wedding clothes so fine,
Spare a thought for this empty life
That you left so far behind.

Look into my dark eyes
And there you may find
A fearful, haunted passage-way
Into my troubled mind.
Fear, rejection, helplessness,
Each has left its mark,
Like fleeting ghosts of memories
That dance there in the dark.

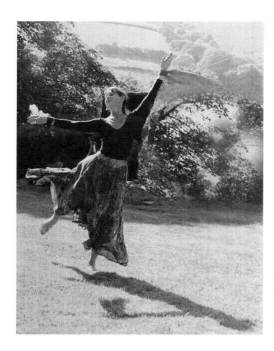

'Trees

That Have

Stood For a
Thousand
Years'

There is an unfortunate tendency within human nature not to appreciate the good things in life until they are under threat, or in many cases, until they have all but disappeared. A bout of sickness tends to increase our appreciation of good health. A brush with death makes us suddenly aware of what a truly amazing gift life is. The number of times I have moped about, nursing a throbbing tooth, only to forget, once the problem has been dealt with, to be thankful for the delicious experience of painlessness. It was not until the very hour that my father died that it dawned on me what a tremendous impact he had had upon my thinking, my perceptions and my values. My entire world-view had been unconsciously shaped by his influence, and suddenly, it was too late to thank him.

It goes without saying that, for good or ill, parents have a considerable impact upon the attitudes and perceptions of their children. A less widely acknowl-edged fact is that the reverse is also true! Although I dedicate this book to the memory of my parents, I am also eager to make it a tribute of thanks to my children (and of course to my husband) who have taught me infinitely well so many of life's most valuable lessons. Up to this point I have been largely pre-occupied with describing the adventures that these same children have led me into, but now I must take a step back in time, in order to relate yet another extraordinary tale.

I referred earlier to my nightmares. I was around twenty years old when I began experiencing these unsettling visitations. I would wake in the night to find figures standing over me. Usually I just screamed in terror, at which point they vanished, leaving me shaking from head to foot.

These visions increased dramatically as time went by. There were many and varied characters who put in appearances. One of the more alarming was a violent woman with piercing eyes and long red flowing hair, who came run-ning straight at me with an enormous javelin. Then there was the 'silent knight' who stood beside my bed in full armour, his visor pulled down over his face; and a white haired, white-clad woman with a wreath of ivy encircling her head. I saw strange, incongruous things: a hand floating above me, a black cat, a grave covered with brightly coloured flowers, a woman silently bending over me, peering at me. Occasionally they turned up in groups, several at a time.

Many years earlier, when I was away dancing in a show, my dead grandmoth-er appeared to me, dressed all in black. I was awakened out of my sleep to find her standing in my room, offering me a bunch of vivid red and white flowers (my mother had always been very superstitious about these being an omen of ill fortune). I found myself in the middle of the room, just about to take the flowers, when I realized what I was doing. I screamed. The vision disap-peared, but when I rang home the next day, I learned that my mother was very ill. Years later I discovered that she had been suffering from depression and had taken an overdose that night.

Of course, I received prayer many times for these unnerving encounters, but although they responded for a while, the visions inevitably came creeping back. In 1983 I accompanied a friend to a meeting where a visiting minister was speaking. Out of the blue came the announcement that there was some-one in the room who suffered from night horrors. I kept quiet at first, think-ing some other person might be in need of help, but when the appeal was made three times and nobody responded, I made my way reluctantly to the front. The speaker took one look at me and asked if I was aware that there was a history of witchcraft in my family. I replied that, although I had no direct knowledge of the fact, I suspected that this was quite probably so. Very humbly he confessed that he was unable to help, but advised me to seek out someone experienced in this area; a task that was to take me another seven years!

As time passed, my nights became more and more troubled. The disturbances diversified into varying degrees of vision, nightmare and sheer horror. Usually the apparitions would slowly change shape and slither out of the window. On one occasion I went to bed, leaving Dimitri watching a late-night film on TV. An hour or so later I woke up, and feeling Dimitri lying beside me, I turned over to see if he, too, was awake. I shall never forget the shock horror of what I saw. Dimitri was nowhere in sight, but there beside me lay a little, shrivelled, wizened old man, whose name I instantly recognized as Death. My skin creeps when I recall the look on his skull-like face.

Gradually the nightmares took on an even more sinister pattern. They were as indescribable in horror as my previous out-of-this-world experience of meeting Jesus in the garden, had been in spiritual wonder. To write about them is difficult for that reason.

Almost every night I would wake to find myself shut into a small, enclosed room, with three other people. One was Dimitri, but the other two were complete strangers. There was no way out, and it suddenly dawned on me that all the events of my life, thus far, had been channelled, as if by some unseen hand, to bring me to this crucial moment. I had been horribly tricked, trapped, and hopelessly abandoned to my fate. What now lay before me was infinitely worse than mere death; that, or annihilation, would have been a welcome end by comparison. The one door in this small, cell-like room led into what I can only describe as a black abyss, a living hell. But in all truth I could never convey the overwhelming sense of horror it inspired in me.

And to think that my own husband had deceived me so dreadfully, and had been an accomplice in the conspiracy! Poor Dimitri was attacked many a night as I fought and clawed at the tricksters. Scornfully, I ignored his cries about it only being another of my dreams. The scoundrel!

As Dylan says, *'Trees that have stood for a thousand years suddenly will fall'.* (11) At the appointed time, institutions or mind-sets that seem as staunch and enduring as an English oak come crashing to the ground. I will now describe how I was finally set free from the torment of these recurring nightmares. But before I launch into this bizarre story, I will first attempt to clarify my personal convictions on the subject of such encounters.

It is my belief that much vital truth is conveyed to us in mythological, symbolic form. The myth, the legend, the archetype, is the fruit containing the seed of fundamental truth, intrinsic to our humanity. We refer glibly to such primeval icons as The Tree of the Knowledge of Good and Evil, and speak of modern technological development as being of the 'fruit' of that tree, bearing both good and evil consequences. Yet what do we really mean by this? I can't help feeling that such mysterious depictions often correspond to rich archetypal realities, and like the parables of Christ, partly reveal yet at the same time partly conceal, a deeper spiritual meaning. Life appears to be full of these half-hidden, gem-like provocations that echo mystically in the deep places of our hearts. Surely the pearl of truth they carry could not be conveyed to us in mere didactic terms. The Spirit of Life invariably clothes life's mysteries in tangible, recognizable forms, which even the simplest of minds can comprehend. Yet the imagery that is used gently pulls at our heartstrings, whispering of deeper truths that cannot be grasped by solely rational, logical means.

Bearing all this in mind, I am not entirely sure what I understand by terms like 'demonic activity' or 'spirit being'. I believe such things exist, but could it not also be the case that, in many instances, psychic phenomena originates in the depths of the unconscious mind? Or like the archetypes, is an extension of a collective, universal, unseen reality? I by no means wish to interpret the vision of my grandmother as a visitation from the dark side, and for similar reasons I hesitate to use the accepted Christian terminology. Like the totem pole, the words or descriptions with which we clothe our experiences often end up replacing the realities they symbolize. However, for the sake of simplicity, I will now go on to use these same terms as I relate this extraordinary tale.

+ + + + + + + + + + + +

It is summer 1990. We are currently living with our family in Wadebridge, North Cornwall. We have decided to pay a visit to our old fellowship at Tremore. On arriving at the manor, we discover that Dr. Adams is taking a break that day. Instead of her usual teaching there is to be a visiting speaker, a certain Malcolm Theobald who, it soon becomes apparent, is something of an authority on the occult.

Malcolm gave a very interesting talk, and after the meeting I decided to ask if he and his wife, Margaret, might be able to offer some advice regarding my night traumas. A meeting was arranged for the following Wednesday evening.

A few days later Dimitri and I made our way once again to the manor, and not really daring to hope for too much, we were ushered into a small study for our interview. Malcolm began by explaining a little about spiritual associations within a family line, and blood covenants, sometimes made by our ancestors, in years gone by. He showed us how these can remain over a family line for a specific number of generations; the blood covenants of occultism being counterfeits of that one, true and ultimate blood covenant made for us by Christ, which is infinitely supreme in power. He then moved on to speak about a specific spiritual influence which he believed could be at the root of my troubles.

The moment he mentioned of this, something strange began happening to me. Gradually, Malcolm's voice receded into the background. The room took on a sinister look as panic swept over me. Strange thoughts and pictures began racing through my head. I could hardly breathe. I went limp all over. My vision blacked out as my head flopped onto my chest. However, I was still fully conscious. In fact I seemed to have a kind of double consciousness; for in that moment I had been gripped by the horrifying realization that the nightmare, which had been troubling me for so long, was now becoming a reality before my very eyes.

.............I found myself in a small enclosed room with three other people. One was Dimitri, the two others, virtual strangers. It seemed that the spiritual power which had identified itself with me all these years had suddenly become aware that, during the course of its life, an unseen hand had been guiding it to this point. There was no way out; before this oppressive spirit stood the doorway to an eternity of blackness, a living hell.

With my mind in turmoil I gripped the sides of my chair, moaning in an effort to break free from the physical incapacity which had taken hold of me. I longed to make a dash for freedom, but struggled with myself to take a position of faith, believing that I had been divinely led to this crucial moment.

Malcolm stood up and took control of the situation. He began emphatically quoting from the book of Revelation about overcoming evil by the sacrificial blood of the Lamb. A huge mental struggle ensued. I felt as if the spirit was a kind of mother to me. It had been a part of me for so long, and in the sense that it had sought to protect itself, it had protected me too. When Malcolm spoke harshly to it, commanding it to leave, I felt like a traitor. I began confusing it with my own mother, seeing pictures of her pleading, pitiful face before my eyes.

Although I was unable to communicate any of this inner turmoil, Margaret Theobald had a word of knowledge, a revelation. She suggested that there was a link, like an umbilical cord, attaching me to the spirit. Verbally they proceeded to cut the cord, while the vision of my mother's face became ever more pitiful.

I remember a sweet fragrance filling the room, the fragrance of the anointing oil. I began to panic as my thoughts raced out of control. Perhaps I was being duped, brainwashed by the use of some strange potion!

Eventually, after a prolonged struggle, I began to feel a sense of release, as well as exhaustion! At last I could see through all the confusion. All those disturbed nights, and it wasn't even my nightmare! The Theobalds, Dimitri and I spent some time discussing and severing past links with the occult. I was told that I would feel a little strange for a few days while I readjusted. I found this to be exactly so, and felt quite exhausted for a time.

That night I was awakened out of my sleep, not by a nightmare, but by a deep sense of peace and tranquility. I fancied, too, that I could smell that fragrance again. Contentedly I drifted back to sleep, happy in the knowledge that my night traumas had finally been dealt with, and that the worst dream of all had been fulfilled in the strangest and most unexpected of ways.

In the months that followed, I was eager to share the story of my dramatic release on two counts: firstly, to communicate to others the reality and power of the unseen world, and secondly, out of a desire to encourage other possible sufferers in the understanding that they are not without hope. My enthusiasm was soon thwarted, however, by the realization that, to most people my experience sounded too far-fetched for them to take me seriously. Thankfully my family did, and it was my eldest son who responded with the words, "Mum you should write a book!" I accepted this as divine prompting and rose to the challenge!

Greatly encouraged as I was by this unexpected turn of events, it was with some disappointment that I found myself still as bound as ever by my obligations in relation to 'the long white ones' of my childhood. It goes without saying that I regarded these phantoms as mere figments of the imagination, but their rules, particularly concerning hand washing, now nearly drove me to distraction. I decided the only way to cope with the problem was to accept that this was an unfortunate but unavoidable part of my make-up. After all, nobody else need ever know about my ever-increasing list of secret compulsions.

We are told that God's ways are past finding out. Certainly there are many inconsistencies in life which tend to leave us baffled. I was so happy to be free from nightmares, thrilled by the almost unfathomable way in which my release had come about, and amazed at the complexity of the spiritual aspect of creation. I was reminded yet again of that very early morning, long ago, when my father had called me into the garden to watch the dew falling. That chance happening of shared wonder had become, for me, another of those cherished memories which are both fascinating, purely through the manifestation of natural laws, yet at the same time seem to echo mystical truths of heavenly things.

The Holy Spirit of the scriptures is frequently likened to *'the dew upon Mount Hermon'*, which is *'as the anointing oil, dripping from the head of the high priest, even to the hem of his garments…'*(12); the high priest of the Old Testament being a type and foreshadow of Christ. In early pre-Christian times, this same Spirit was depicted as the divine feminine; or as the wind, a river in flood, oil or fire. God can reveal himself to us in a multiplicity of guises; we sense his stirrings, long after him, and delight to feel his effect upon our lives. I have used here the currently popular patriarchal terminology, but increasingly I sense the need to perceive the Godhead as androgynous. Unless we honour and respect the earth as the sacred womb from which we come, and refrain from the rape and abuse of our very life source, there seems little hope of our own, or our planet's survival.

Every aspect of creation speaks to us, in some way, about the One who brought it into being. The psalmist proclaims, *'The heavens declare the glory of God'*.(13) The Great I Am has set this beautiful world within a rhythmic pattern. The times, days, seasons; our bodies, lives and work are ordered by the pulsating rhythm of creation. Like any other repetitive function, this can serve either as a basic formula for liberation, or equally, as a snare. It is my belief that the heart of the created order beats for freedom, rather like the time signature of a musical score. The 'one-two-three, one-two-three' of a waltz might seem remarkably repetitive, but the skilled composer uses this basic framework upon which to hang countless variations for his work, producing marvellously inspiring atmospheres and dramatic changes of mood in the creation of his music. In our desire for security, and our inappropriate application of tradition, we can so easily fall into the trap of using the liberating rhythm of life to become mundane creatures of habit. The church has to be the biggest culprit and number one example of this discrepancy. How incredible that the most ancient, mystical, paradoxical collection of writings, so unfathomably rich in wisdom, symbolism and history, should be presented as a boring, outdated compilation of irrelevant fables, intermittently interspersed with a long list of 'thou shalt nots'. Little wonder Eastern mysticism and the cult of the New Age appear more attractive to so many.

Surely we would do better to leave aside our pat answers, and rather immerse ourselves in the unfathomable mysteries of life. Portrayed in the book of Proverbs as a woman, Wisdom is said to have existed before the formation of the primeval dust of earth. She is the goddess Sophia, *'the master craftsperson'* who playfully danced at the birth of the planets. It is she who calls to men from the high hills, beside the way where the paths meet, urging them to seek after her, and join her in the dance of life.(14)

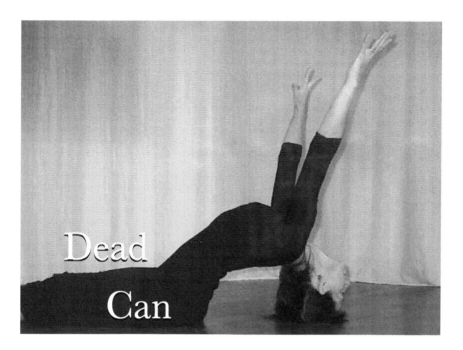

Dead Can

Dance

Shortly after our move to North Cornwall, Dimitri and I decided it would be a good idea to start bi-monthly arts meetings for disillusioned artists like ourselves. People travelled from the far reaches of the county, as well as a few brave souls who actually crossed the River Tamar, and met in our living room where we ate nice food, aired our grievances, and generally offered encouragement to each other. After a number of these sessions, Dimitri suggested that perhaps we might venture to do something a little more constructive, and indeed we did succeed in putting on a number of cabaret evenings at The Indian King, a local arts centre. But, for the most part, our companions were content with eating and talking, which admittedly was very pleasant if not entirely ground breaking in its results.

Occasionally we were able to invite professional speakers to our gatherings. Ian Traynor, a member of the Arts Centre Group in London, proved particularly helpful. He joined us one month and gave a very beneficial talk. Ian went on to encourage Dimitri and myself to become involved on a national scale, and the following year, handed over to Dimitri the job of arts coordinator for the Cross Rhythms Festival in Okehampton. Over the course of the next eight years, the Arts and Theatre Tent was built up from virtually nothing, to a hive of creativity. Of course, this was a great opportunity for me, as it created a platform for my choreography, and also brought me into contact with the many other performers whom I was working alongside. For several years I worked with Mary Palmer, a poet from Bath. This was an excellent experience, not only of dancing to the spoken word, but the idea of serving another person's art form, endeavouring to enhance and illuminate the ethos of the poem, all added a new dimension to my use of movement.

Dimitri's work as speaker and arts facilitator rapidly began to grow. He was asked to take on a similar task at a festival in the Midlands, and the following year we were both invited to speak, exhibit and perform in Ireland. This, in turn, resulted in many more invitations to share ideas and coordinate events. Dimitri was elected to sit on the board of the London based Arts Centre Group and also to take on the role of regional coordinator. He later embarked upon a quest involving the rediscovery of his Greek roots, which led to a complete change of style in his work. He began painting large, very modern icons in vibrant colours, and was offered exhibitions in many cathedrals up and down the country. It was when I danced in the Midlands that something truly life-changing occurred. But this I will come to a little later

Many significant things now began opening up for us by way of performances, exhibitions, festivals, speaking engagements, and in the drawing together of other artists from around the UK. But, as so often happens, just as the green light shows and everything seems to be heading right on course, enormous obstacles appear, for no other apparent reason than to block the way. This has happened, to our utter frustration, time and time again.

✦✦✦✦✦✦✦✦✦✦✦✦

There was a time when I worried a lot about the fact that my parents would one day grow old and die. In reality, the older they became the less likelihood there seemed of this ever happening. They were so active and both enjoyed life so much, I began to doubt I would out-live them! My father's sudden death, in April 1995, came as a complete shock, in spite of his eighty-nine years. Never before had I experienced such grief and devastating emotional pain. As for my mother, after sixty-five years of marriage, I cannot imagine how she coped with her loss. In spite of her good health, she only survived him by eighteen months. My two brothers, my sister and I rallied together and did our best to support her during that intervening time. With six people still living at home (seven during the holidays when Jude returned) it was difficult for me, travelling to and from St. Austell where she lived. My mother came to stay with us for increasingly long periods of time until, eventually, she moved in permanently. For some months now we had been renting a spacious bungalow on the outskirts of Wadebridge. I was so thankful that we were, once again, able to accommodate such a large number of people.

I truly wanted to help my Mum and make her remaining years as happy as possible. Although she was as good as gold, I believe I was pretty much a failure. It was so frustrating never having a moment to myself. In order to choreograph dances it is imperative for me to be alone. I need to improvise, to be free to abandon myself to the ethos of the music, and to intuitively feel my way through a piece as the movements mould themselves into the sounds. Although we were such a house-full, there had been times throughout the day when people were at work or school and I could do this. Not any longer!

There was one morning in particular, just a few months after my father's death, when the reality of her bereavement seemed to hit my mother afresh, and she cried inconsolably. Distraught, and still dealing with my own grief, I looked desperately for a way to help her.

Before long a knock sounded at the front door. There on the doorstep stood Andy Smith, the pastor of our local church. He was not usually in the habit of cold calling. With an almost apologetic air he began explaining that, whilst he could be quite mistaken, he thought he had felt some kind of divine prompting to visit us that morning. Thankfully, I invited him to come and meet my Mum.

Immediately, my mother began pouring her heart out to him. But before she had got very far, a second knock sounded. This time it was the assistant pastor, apparently having had the same prompting. He stared in surprise at Andy standing in my kitchen! Within a very short time, both ministers were leading my grief-stricken mother, in prayer, to a saving relationship with Jesus. Amazingly, there followed a swift transformation from hopeless grief to sheer joy.

"It's a miracle!" she repeated over and over again; and then, turning to Andy, a note of anxiety in her voice, "But will he know? Will my husband know what's happened to me?" We assured her that, according to scripture, there is joyful celebration in heaven whenever one repentant sinner turns to God. We were certain that my Dad would be joining in the party!

My mother went on to her higher calling not so very many months after this episode. The events of that morning were, for me, not only an answer to my prayers, but a confirmation of the all-pervasive love of God, bringing comfort and healing at a time of grief and loss. I am so very glad to know that the pain of my parents' separation is now over, and that some day we will all be reunited.

In the meantime, during the months that my mother remained with us, I was finding the pressures and restrictions upon my life impossibly difficult to cope with. With hindsight, I wish with all my heart I had known how short a time my dear old Mum had left. Gradually she ate less and less, slept more and more, until one November morning her heart finally gave up beating. Grief swept in once again, mingled with shock, remorse and guilt at the terrible frustration I had been feeling. When my mother died, something inside me died too.

One by one, over the course of the next few months, our children began to drift away. Jude left for Southampton to study graphics. Daniel, who had completed his foundation year at Falmouth, was accepted at Winchester School of Art. Seth moved to St. Austell, and Demi, who had been staying with us temporarily, found other accommodation. Only Lydia remained at home. A short while before, it had seemed as if the whole world depended on me. Now, for the first time in almost thirty years, I felt superfluous! My creativity shrivelled up. Dimitri had arranged for me to dance in Bath the following May, and I was booked to perform at The Cross Rhythms Festival in July. I had no new work to contribute and I certainly had no desire to produce any. I decided that I would somehow summon up the energy to fulfil these two obligations and then give up dancing ......forever.

A time of emptiness followed. I found myself engulfed by a creative drought that drained me of any desire to even think about dancing. Several months passed. May came and went. I managed to get through my performance at The Bath Festival quite successfully. It was a first time for me in this area, so I was able to get away with using pieces from my existing repertoire. But the prospect of performing at Cross Rhythms, where I had danced on so many previous occasions, still daunted me terribly. Then, one day, a member of The Elastic Band happened to lend us a new music album by a group with the marvellous name, 'Dead Can Dance'. Their music was deep, rich and evocative, in a style I later learnt is described as 'world music'. One track in particular, a woman's wailing lament, stirred something deep inside me. Was it possible that I could choreograph just one last piece? A dance that expressed a woman's anguish at coming to terms with an ageing body? I decided to try.

✝ ✝ ✝ ✝ ✝ ✝ ✝ ✝ ✝ ✝ ✝ ✝ ✝

Unravelling and deciphering one's own artwork is rather like interpreting one's dreams. Once inspiration takes hold of me, I become captivated in an intense whirl of excitement, yet frequently with only a vague impression of what the final portrayal will be. It is sometimes weeks later, even after performing the piece several times, that the penny finally drops and the full picture emerges.

As my new dance progressed, I realized the interpretation went much deeper than merely the concept of ageing, although this remained an integral part of the main theme. It became expressive of many of the emotions and yearnings of early childhood, yet linked inextricably to my own experience as a mother; the joys and sorrows of bearing with a young family over the years.

It is my belief that deep within every man there lives a little boy, but within every little girl there lives a woman. Looking back over my childhood, I have often wondered at the deep stirrings of maternal instinct within me, even in my earliest recollections. A sense of love and womanhood spilled into me from my own mother, and was eagerly awaiting a time in the distant future when this might flow on into successive generations. Years later, when as a young adult I fell in love for the first time, I was astonished to discover that those early awakenings were actually associated with this delightful, yet painful state of affairs! How much greater was the subsequent revelation, that this enigmatic condition known as 'being in love', was merely a shadow, a foretaste of a far deeper mystery: the mystery of Christ and his church, and of the 'animus' as revealed by the psychologist Jung. To my amazement, the dance was becoming **'a reflection on womanhood'**.

I do not wish to appear in any way unfeeling towards women who, for whatever reasons, do not become mothers. I am always so glad that there are those who choose to remain childless. They compensate for the greedy ones, like me, who don't know when to stop. As for those women who are unable to conceive, my heart truly goes out to them. But the essential attributes of womanhood are not restricted solely to service within the family. However, it is the role of 'mother' which, in our modern society, is becoming increasingly undermined.

It is a sad fact that, today, raising a family is frequently regarded as of secondary importance to having a career, or a well-paid job. Yet motherhood is an enormous privilege, a gift. Children are only children for a relatively short period of time, although it seems an eternity to them (and often to us!) It is an unfortunate trend in today's world that so many small children are being denied that valuable period of development in the nest, while Mum has little option but to pursue the all important task of holding down a job. Relational and parental skills are not learnt academically but by example, and above all, by being needed, cherished and loved within the natural environment of the home. If our little ones mean more to us than all the riches in the world, how unfortunate it is that parents are under such pressure to sacrifice those precious childhood years for mere financial gain. In times past I too have almost apologetically referred to myself as 'only a mum and a housewife', when in fact, that is the most important job a woman could ever hope to do. Mighty trees grow from the tiniest of seeds. The family is, after all, the foundational basis of society.

But to return to my dance! In the second act I work with a length of black cloth, at times completely obscuring myself from the audience's view. It was not until I had actually performed the piece on stage for the first time that I grasped the full implication of this. The cloth represents those things that, on the face of it, seem to hinder and restrict us. Yet frequently it is the outworking of those same limitations that can enrich our experience of life, leading us on to greater freedom and independence. I refer to such qualities as loyalty, perseverance, faithfulness. All of which go hand in hand with activities like study, training, even bringing up a family!

Working these ideas through choreographically, soaking up these impressions of the strength and power of womanhood, and in particular of motherhood, I found fresh ideas forming in my mind: ways in which these fundamental yet vital issues might be highlighted through movement. But if nothing else, I knew I had come alive again. In my recent wanderings through that barren wilderness of grief, I had finally stumbled upon springs of water to refresh and revitalize my soul!

It was several months after this unexpected burst of inspiration that my imagination was once more stirred into action; this time by an album of Israeli-style music, entitled Sh'ma Yisrael. The track that especially caught my attention had all kinds of sounds superimposed over it. There was a news bulletin, voices, the sound of scuffling and fighting, children wailing. In the background the shofar, the temple ram's horn, could be heard calling the nation to attention. The over-all theme was the return of the Jewish people to their homeland after a two thousand year exile.

Inspired once more, I set to work. By the second day of my involvement with the new dance, it began to dawn on me that this was not, after all, an isolated and separate piece of choreography, but was, to my astonishment, linked to my previous work. The theme of motherhood was simply being moved onto a much bigger picture.

'Deep calls to deep at the sound of your cataracts'.(15) I felt I was being stirred up and alerted to a fresh understanding of the origin and birthplace, not only of Judaism, but also of Christianity and Islam. Those two brothers, Jacob and Esau, who are representative of the Jewish and Palestinian nations, continue to struggle together in the womb of their motherland.(16) The failure to recognize their mutual blood ties serving only to heighten the appalling tragedy of this apparently irresolvable conflict.

I once watched a nature programme on TV about a strange reptile called a tree-lizard. This creature has developed an insidious habit of seeking out unattended birds' nests, eating the contents, and then laying its own eggs in place of those just consumed. Then off it creeps, leaving its clutch to be hatched by the unsuspecting parent birds. What a shock when the poor parents eventually discover that they have been nurturing a brood of murderous monsters!

In some ways I fear this same scenario is being re-enacted within Judaism. Certainly the horrors of the holocaust should have taught the world an unforgettable lesson. Yet without forgiveness and reconciliation, the seeds of the spirit of Nazism can so easily live on to be cultivated in our midst (as in the analogy of the obnoxious tree lizard). In both cases the 'chosen race' has ruthlessly sought ascendancy over its own blood brothers; a far cry from the concept of peacemakers inheriting the land. Why is it, I wonder, that so many of Christ's followers are convinced that the Jews are somehow exempt from the Messiah's exhortation to 'love our enemies'? Weren't they the very people he was addressing at the time? As always, there are, in the midst of the atrocities, scores of innocent victims from both camps. And as in the case of the

Palestinian Melkite pastor, Elias Chacour, whose family was mercilessly driven from their ancient Galilean home by occupying Israeli troops in the late 1940s, many Palestinians fully recognize the need for reconciliation in a truly Christian context. One wonders if Israel, like its fore-father of old, will wrestle with the Angel of God for its blessing, and quite what will be the outcome of such a struggle.

✢ ✢ ✢ ✢ ✢ ✢ ✢ ✢ ✢ ✢ ✢ ✢ ✢

As I look back on that barren period following my mother's death, when I came so close to giving up dancing altogether, I seem to see, in my mind's eye, Ezekiel's valley of dry bones.(17) Miraculously, I felt as if new life had been breathed into my shrivelled soul, inspiring me to create one of the most poignant dance series I had ever produced. And in spite of the tragic failure of the Abrahamic races to embrace the radical teaching of their Messiah, those very dry bones, the Jewish people, have been revived, even after the devastation of Hitler's holocaust.

Perhaps it is more than mere coincidence that the original music that so inspired me to dance again was called Dead Can Dance. As well as being applicable to my rebirth into dance, the series that I went on to produce actually became a tribute to my mother's life. She too had once been a dancer. It equally described the final piece of choreography as it slotted into place. I decided to keep this very apt name as the title of the complete work.

What I failed to realize at this point, however, was the surprising way in which this particular theme was to link up with the next chapter in my life.

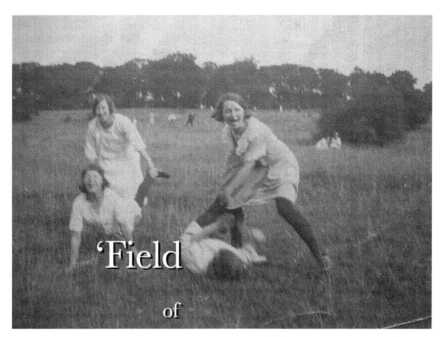

'Field
of
Dreams'

Wheelbarrow race. May Enoch standing right

I referred earlier to a remarkable incident at a festival in the Midlands. In the autumn of 1997 I danced at the Roots and Branches Festival in Dudley Castle, and it was whilst I was here that a tiny seed was sown in my mind. Like most other seeds, it was soon covered over and largely forgotten about. Susie Brock, the wife of a Hawaiian minister, saw me perform my new work, 'Dead Can Dance', although this was before the creation of the final piece, 'Sh'ma Yisrael'. Apparently, she was so deeply moved that she sought me out afterwards and introduced herself to me. We talked for a while and shared a little about our experiences. Susie then announced that she had a 'word' for me. She was certain that something new was about to open up for me regarding my dancing, but she had no idea what this could be.

Of course, that was all very interesting, but one can't spend one's entire life waiting for unlikely things to happen. And after all, nothing out of the ordinary did happen, for several months. Then one day in May of the following year, about six weeks after my involvement with 'Sh'ma', I received a phone call from the wife and manager of London-based musician, Paul Heyman. Paul had also performed at the Dudley Festival the previous autumn. His act had followed mine, and we had spent a short time together discussing the possibility of booking him for the Arts Tent at Cross Rhythms. Paul is a messianic Jew, and a wonderfully accomplished, virtuoso electric violinist. He had recently left Helen Shapiro's touring band in order to develop his work as a solo artist. Previous to this he had played with the orchestra of London's Festival Ballet and so was quite at home working with dancers. Now his wife, Jan, was asking if I would be willing to choreograph a series of dances to Paul's album, Israel's Passion. I was invited to work with him at Glastonbury Abbey in July, and following this at The Birmingham Festival. Later that year, if all went to plan, we would perform together at The Edinburgh Festival. Not surprisingly, I agreed!

It was decided that we would use Cross Rhythms as a testing-ground for the combination of our work. I immediately began experimenting, adding hints of Israeli dancing to my already fairly unique style. Over the years I have developed a very dramatic medium, after the style of Martha Graham, but using the basic techniques and pathways of classical ballet. Fortunately, Paul's music is very varied in content and we perform works ranging from classical to contemporary, light-hearted to dramatic, character to rock-and-roll. Initially I had a huge struggle with guilt. The luxury of allotting myself several hours each day for choreography made me feel incredibly selfish. I rapidly learnt to overcome this problem!

Once creativity is unleashed it does tend to take over one's life. All sorts of new ideas for further work of my own, in addition to the arrangements for Paul, began flooding in. My brain was fairly vibrating as it struggled to cope with all the new material that was being committed to memory day after day.

Years earlier, when as a little girl I had dreamed of becoming a ballerina, I had always suspected that there was something far deeper, and more mystical, to be discovered through the medium of dance, even than fame or success, attractive though these were. I sensed that, encapsulated in my desire to dance was a wonderful secret that was waiting to be unveiled.

Life is full of riddles that can neither be touched with the hand nor apprehended by the eye, although they dwell within each of us, and are manifest only by the fruit that is born from them. And this fruit is also enigmatic in nature, requiring a deal of fathoming, like the symbolism of allegory. In recent years I have discovered that, for me, the hidden power of dance lies in the thrill of sharing shadows, simple parables that whisper great truths.

From my earliest schooldays, I remember being fascinated by the story of Jephthah's daughter, a young Hebrew girl who made the fatal mistake of dancing out to greet her father on his victorious return from a huge tribal battle, only to learn that she was to become the next human sacrifice. As I contemplated this tragic and unnecessary waste of a young life, I began to see a parallel emerging in certain aspects of our present-day belief patterns.

With the benefit of hindsight, it is not difficult to see that the Hebrew people of old had retained many of the barbaric traditions of their pre-Abrahamic heritage, and had returned to the once common practice of child sacrifice (even Abraham willingly sent his firstborn to perish in the desert, but was thankfully spared the trouble of slaying his second) all the while believing that they were acting in obedience to their God. A few thousand years later, the Christian church appears to be operating under the same delusion. While confessing to be 'in the world but not of it', its dreams and aspirations often disclose a desire to integrate, and identify with, the very system that it seeks to shun. In effect, modern culture acts rather like a whirlpool, sucking unsuspecting victims into a life-style that revolves chiefly around the pursuit of worldly success. The true cost of our service to this insatiable god of consumerism, who has cast his all-encompassing, invisible web over western society, is impossible to calculate. In effect, we are sacrificing our very lives, our children, and our posterity.

As I reflected on these ideas, possibilities for a future dance series were conceived in my imagination. But the ways in which the scenes emerge and the music comes to me, all seem to be quite out of my hands. Invariably it has been Jude who has unwittingly supplied me with the most appropriate, if unlikely, music for my choreography.

I have danced The Lament of Jephthah's Daughter many times, but perhaps the most thrilling of all was at the Christian Artists Seminars in Holland. This is an annual event, funded by the EU, in which artists from all over Europe are invited to take part. Many well-known musicians, singers, visual artists, dancers, dramatists, film producers, and indeed artistes of all genres, have benefited and received encouragement over the years, from this prestigious and inspiring festival. Frankly, I was terrified, and spent my first day at the centre in floods of tears. The standard was so unbelievably high! Here artists are invited to perform, exhibit, speak about their work, or take seminars. Not, as all too frequently happens, because they are pop idols or TV stars (although many are, in their own countries), but rather because of the quality and content of their work. Consequently there is always a refreshing mix of seasoned celebrities and lesser-known artists. I was working alongside Springs Dance Company; all excellent dancers, and all at least twenty-five years younger than I am! Euphemistically speaking, I was reluctant to perform!

The response to my performance, however, was staggering. I was thrilled when Sir Leen La Rivière, the director and mastermind behind the organization, came to speak with me afterwards, kissing my hand and congratulating me on my work. The admiration expressed by all the other artists was overwhelming. There was one lovely lady, herself a distinguished opera singer called Martha-Jo Smith, an American currently living in Oslo, who was particularly encouraging. Martha-Jo really helped me to believe in myself and in the quality of my performance. She offered much sound advice on the way forward, as she was eager for my work to be promoted throughout major venues in London, but unfortunately the precarious nature of our lifestyle has largely hindered us from acting upon her counsel.

Meanwhile, the work with Paul Heyman continued to expand with the launching of his second album. The combination of our particular styles of music and dance blend so remarkably well, that we have gone on to perform and tour together a great deal. After years of endeavouring to suppress my creativity, simply through lack of time and opportunity, this sudden stimulation and demand for choreography caused a positive eruption of inspiration and ideas. I soon built up a substantial repertoire of my own work, quite apart from the dances I had created for Paul. It was not long before I began receiving invitations to perform this new work in venues all over the UK, as well in Europe.

In the year 2000, Paul and I took part in Cliff Richard's Gala Performance at Glastonbury Abbey. It was a great honour to share a stage with such artists as Noel Richards, Graham Kendrick and Rick Wakeman, as well as with the super-star himself. I had the privilege of dancing three solos, accompanied by Paul and the All Souls Orchestra, a huge, sixty-strong affair. The immensity of the stage, the dazzling laser lights, not to mention the multitude in the audience, all sent my legs to jelly and made me wish momentarily that I was back home in cosy little Wadebridge!

If all this sounds wildly exciting, well, in some ways it is, but only during the high times. Such a lifestyle often involves either a mountain top, or a 'mountain-topped', experience. In other words, you can be on top of the mountain one day, and the next day *it* will be on top of *you!* Dimitri and I struggle constantly with financial problems. We have never recovered, in that sense, from the loss of our home. Believe me; it requires an enormous amount of determination, hard work and single-mindedness to remain at performance level after one's fiftieth birthday! It is essential that I regularly spend time working out, choreographing new pieces and rehearsing my existing repertoire. More recently I have concentrated on building up my work as a teacher, but although I enjoy having an input into the lives of others, seeing people develop technically and artistically, my heart will always be in creating and performing. When the time comes for me to face the final curtain, I would far sooner turn my hand to writing than to teaching. It seems that I am destined (or determined) to remain a penniless artist for the rest of my days!

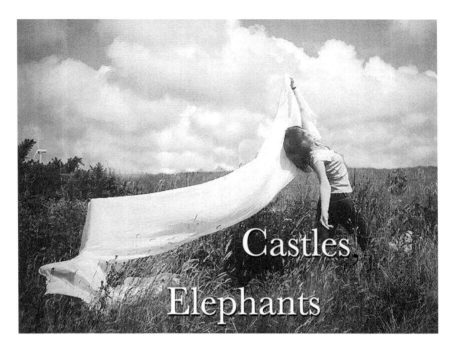

Castles
Elephants
and Irishmen

I have found it reassuring, as well as enlightening, to read the biographies of several dancers of the Diaghilev era, and to discover that they, like so many early pioneers of the arts, frequently found themselves working in less than desirable circumstances, often being misunderstood, ridiculed and rejected. Vaslav Nijinsky, even after receiving world-wide acclaim as the greatest male dancer of all time, succeeded in bringing the entire audience of The Champs Elysées Theatre to its feet, not in rapturous applause as was his normal habit, but with cat-calls, frenzied shouting and wild abuse, following the première of his revolutionary choreographic work, Le Sacre du Printemps. Isadora Duncan was forced to dance barefoot amongst a shower of tin-tacks (probably because her feet were not the only parts of her anatomy that were revealed as she danced!) During the war years several former stars of the Ballets Russes were reduced to performing in run down theatres, performing dubious pieces, just to keep a roof over their heads and food on the table.

Although I now perform work with a far greater depth than anything I had previously been involved in, I dance less in the comfort of major theatres and more often in cathedrals, churches, art centres, smaller theatres and festivals. It is not unheard of for event organizers to overlook the need for dancers to warm up before a performance. Occasionally, I even have to haggle in order to get a proper space rehearsal prior to the show. I am frequently expected to spend long periods of time between spots, cooped up in a chilly changing area the size of a broom-cupboard…and then appear on stage as lithe, supple and fresh as if I had just emerged from the classroom!

Such thoughts take me back to the day we arrived, together with the Heymans, in Dublin airport at the start of our Ireland tour. We were met by Rodney, a retired architect; an amiable, extraordinarily generous fellow, who had undertaken to arrange and finance our entire stay in the lovely Emerald Isle. Rodney took us to meet our hosts, an elderly couple who lived in a beautiful old-fashioned farmhouse, situated in a rambling valley deep in the countryside of County Wicklow. After a sumptuous meal (the Irish are clearly under the impression that we English are under-nourished), we were taken to view the venue where our first performance was due to take place the following day. Just as he was about to usher us inside, Rodney coughed a little hesitantly. "Er, about the stage," he began (I had been assured during an earlier telephone conversation that this met with my specified requirements of a minimum 12ft x 12ft area) "It's very large but……well, does it matter that it's on three levels?"

Thank goodness Rodney was in such an appropriate profession! He knew exactly where to buy all the necessary materials. Next day both he and Dimitri set to work, and between them they succeeded in constructing a perfectly adequate wooden stage, just hours before the concert, completely overlaying the precarious, three-tiered affair of part stone, part wood and part carpet, that I would otherwise have been faced with!

During the second week of the tour, we were scheduled to work in Belfast. Again our hosts, and in fact everyone we met, were overwhelmingly friendly and hospitable.....except when we were out on the road. It never failed to surprise us that every time we stopped a passer-by in order to ask the way, we were eyed with suspicion and pointed in totally the opposite direction! On one particularly frustrating day, when we were trying to locate the venue for that evening's event, we found ourselves being sent on such a wild goose chase that it took nothing less than the law to sort out our predicament. We were finally escorted to our destination by a group of four policemen on motorbikes. It seemed that they were the only people willing to help us! A few days later, it was pointed out to us that our vehicle, a people-carrier which Rodney had kindly hired for our travel requirements, had a republican registration number. No wonder we struck terror into the hearts of all those poor people whom we encountered on the streets of Belfast!

During this same tour, Jan Heyman caught the most dreadful cold. Spending long hours cooped up together on the road, Dimitri and I inevitably went down with it. We arrived back in England in a rather miserable state, both with sore throats, streaming noses, and feeling decidedly out of sorts. We met up with the Heymans a couple of days later in Bangor, North Wales. Our next port of call was to be the Spring Harvest Festival at Pwllheli. It had been a long day. It was also my birthday. As we entered the travel lodge where we were to spend the night, we were greeted by Paul's rendering of 'Happy Birthday to You' on the violin. Characteristically, Dimitri had forgotten!

Exhausted after the day's journey, we found our rooms and soon settled down to a welcome night's rest. It was very late. At around 2 a.m., just as I was beginning to drift into a delicious state of unconsciousness, we were woken abruptly by the ringing of our smoke alarm. What, we wondered, could possibly be the reason for this dreadful din? We leapt out of bed and began violently waving arms and newspapers in a fruitless attempt to quell the noise. Dimitri, in exasperation, started jumping up and down, swatting the offending alarm, which was attached to the ceiling. At this point there was a knock on the door. Ah! No doubt a helpful warden had come to our aid. It was Jan, asking anxiously why we hadn't joined the multitude of other pyjama-clad inmates who were now safely assembled outside in the courtyard. Hastily, we pulled on our coats, shuffled into our shoes and fled!

It was freezing that night! My mind immediately conjures up images of frost and fluttering snowflakes, but I think this is probably going too far. After about an hour of shivering nervously in the raw March air, we were at last permitted to re-enter the building. The problem had been identified as a mere electrical fault and not, as we had begun to suspect, the IRA on an exchange visit!

Next morning, our colds not much improved by the antics of the previous night, we set off for Pwllheli; a twenty minute drive away, or so we were told. We soon lost the Heymans, but this didn't present any great problem as our directions were pretty clear. Obviously not clear enough! Looking back, I think that perhaps crossing the Menai Bridge *should* have been a clue, but then again, *I* was navigating, and I'm notoriously unobservant. An hour or so later, suspecting that Welsh minutes were comparable to Cornish miles, or else that we had somehow lost the plot, Dimitri called in at a little village shop.

"Could you tell us where we are?" he enquired, thrusting a map under the shopkeeper's nose and trying not to sound as exasperated as he was feeling. The shop assistant peered at the map for a few seconds and then pointed to the tip of Anglesey. We had almost made it to Holyhead! A few more yards and we'd have been boarding the ferry back to Dublin!

Eventually, after another long drive, we succeeded in finding the festival site. It didn't seem to matter that we were late. Nobody appeared to remember that they had booked us, or that accommodation had been reserved for us. The receptionist and staff had apparently mislaid all information regarding performers. Just a minor hitch!

After a lot of hanging about, profuse apologies were offered on behalf of the management and we were finally escorted to our chalets, and later to the performance area for a sound check. I found, to my relief, that the stage on this occasion was large and perfectly adequate. It was heartening to see the crowds come pouring in for our late-night show. We got off to a good start. As usual, Paul played the first number alone and I joined him for the second. At the end of this piece a steward appeared, striding purposefully onto the stage and grabbing the mike. To our astonishment he ordered everyone to evacuate the building. It seemed that our lives were in jeopardy. A suspected bomb had been discovered in our midst. Oh please! Not the IRA again!

I think in the end it turned out to be nothing more life-threatening than a stray rucksack that had aroused the suspicions of an over-excited passer-by. We did eventually manage to finish our performance, but I guess it turned out to be more of an early-morning show than the late-night spot we had planned!

✢ ✢ ✢ ✢ ✢ ✢ ✢ ✢ ✢ ✢ ✢ ✢ ✢

Whenever we are away on tour, our accommodation arrangements are left in the capable hands of the event organizers. On the whole this has turned out very well for us. Sometimes we stay at a B&B, occasionally at a hotel, but more often we are welcomed into people's homes, fed lavishly and made to feel like royalty for the duration of our stay.

However, the first time that I danced at the Dudley festival (prior to my teaming up with Paul Heyman) we opted to stay at Dimitri's mother's house in Birmingham, although on this particular occasion she was away in Cyprus. Unfortunately, it was not until late that night, following our first day at the festival, that we discovered our communication system had failed. After driving up and down the Pershore Road (it's a very long road!) half a dozen times or more in the early hours of the morning, in search of missing relatives who we believed to be holding the house-keys, it seemed that we had little option but to abandon this particular plan. But not before we had been pulled over by the law on grounds of suspicious behaviour! Apparently, a police car had been following us as we zoomed, this way and that, occasionally stopping to creep up dark garden paths and peer in at the windows of empty houses. We were asked to tell our story: a tale which sounded increasingly ridiculous as we dribbled explanations about our long drive from Cornwall early that morning, my performance at Dudley Castle, Mother in Cyprus, and the missing key-holder. The policeman responded by demanding a demonstration of Dimitri's ability to walk in a straight line. Satisfied, at least, that we were neither perspective bank robbers nor rolling drunk, we were acquitted. But we were strongly advised against our most recent plan of spending the night in nearby Selley Park. We were warned that this might well result in our being 'rolled over'.

Dimitri and I looked at each other in dismay. What on earth were we to do? Exhausted after the events of the day, I felt I might cheerfully have robbed a whole chain of banks if this could have ensured us a bed for the night and a cup of hot tea. But since the time was well after 2 a.m. such luxuries appeared to be totally out of the question. Not knowing what else to do, we turned in our tracks and headed back towards Dudley.

At around 3 a.m. two very sleepy individuals rolled in to the now familiar driveway that led up to Dudley Castle. There below the castle grounds stood Dudley Zoo, strangely quiet and shrouded in darkness. And it was here, beside the elephant enclosure, accompanied by a mother elephant and her calf that we quietly froze till morning, cramped up in the back of our old estate car. At first light I sidled out of the boot, leaving Dimitri in a state of semi-conscious abandon. Having first paid my respects to my companions in the adjoining pen, I set off to wander the deserted town in search of an open tea-shop; a quest that was to take me another two hours. Dimitri eventually caught up with me, and together we succeeded in finding a little café that served hot tea and toast. Never had such simple fare tasted so good!

By this time I was feeling less like a dancer than a new-age traveller. The weather had turned decidedly chilly that weekend. Autumn had arrived early in the Midlands, whereas back home in Cornwall we had been enjoying a spell of late summer sunshine. In spite of the cold, it turned out to be a pleasant enough day. Dimitri and I had very little to do earlier on. All the best acts were scheduled for the evening, but the ancient castle itself was an interesting place to explore. The venue where I was to dance that night was an area known as 'The Tunnel', a former dungeon, now containing many historical relics including several suits of armour!

As shadows lengthened my temper grew correspondingly shorter. I was hungry! I needed to warm up for my spot. By now my tired body ached so much that I would have given anything to have absconded. In fact, I was quite desperate to find a way out of my commitment. These feelings of rebellion led to my indulging in a large portion of fish and chips (Dudley has an exceptionally good chip shop). By the time I had consumed this feast my dance outfit was feeling uncommonly tight!

But life is full of surprises and sometimes the very thing we dread so terribly turns out to be the biggest blessing of all. I seem to have told this particular anecdote back to front, but had I not danced that night, even in my exhausted, fit-to-bust state, Susie Brock would never have noticed me, and neither would Paul Heyman. Presumably my life would have carried on in much the same way as it had over the past twenty or more years. What a different story I would be telling!

In retrospect, all these little escapades create excellent subject matter for storytelling, especially to our grandchildren, who are probably all under the impression that we are a couple of quaint oddities. I remember returning home after the wettest year ever at Cross Rhythms; we and all our belongings completely covered in mud and dirt. Our children merely shrugged resignedly when they beheld our bedraggled state. Here come Mum and Dad, behaving like a couple of adolescents again!

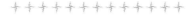

One memorable adventure occurred during a trip to Italy. Having moved to Exeter just a couple of weeks earlier (oh, sad day that we tore ourselves away from beautiful Cornwall in order to be closer to the motor-way!) I was not relishing the prospect of travelling into the unknown. Of course, under normal circumstances I love venturing out to unfamiliar destinations for the purpose of performing, but the recent upheaval of moving house had taken its toll on my energy levels. Also Esteban Antonio, the flamenco guitarist with whom I was scheduled to appear, had pulled out at the last minute.

We set out on our journey from Exeter to Stanstead a day early, for fear of being caught up in congestion on the motorway. We planned to find a cheap B&B close to the airport. The traffic reports on the radio were so horrendous that we soon abandoned any attempt to circum-navigate London via the M25. Since we had several hours to spare, we decided instead to visit our son, Daniel, at his digs in Elephant and Castle.

There was something distinctly déja vu associated with this turn of events. A subliminal link with past experiences involving these large, lumbering, yet endearing beasts, as well as with castles and cramped over-night accommodation in the frozen wastes of V.W. estate cars.......Yes, you've guessed it! After an enormous and totally delicious meal with Dan at the cheapest Chinese restaurant in town, we eventually arrived in Stanstead at around 1.30 a.m. By this time every B&B and travel-lodge was firmly locked up for the night. I was in no mood for adventure but our options were limited, probably non-existent.

Muttering something about the ridiculous concept of a dancer-cum-granny spending the night in the back of a car, with no pillow, blanket, or single item of warmth or comfort, I grudgingly stretched out on the cold, metallic lumpiness of the car floor. And yes, it was *freezing*, in spite of it being July. And no, I didn't sleep a *wink*, even though my suspicions were duly confirmed the following day when, on arriving in Tourin, I discovered I was scheduled to dance that same evening. As it happened, I was so tired that my habitual stage fright was almost entirely over-ruled by exhaustion. Maybe, after all, it wasn't such a bad thing that I had spent so uncomfortable a night!

Our stay in Italy was unforgettable. The Anno Domini Multifestival was held high up in the Alps of Northern Italy, in Oropa, a twelfth century monastery. Our bedroom (we slept in the converted monks' cells) was situated above a deep gorge, with a river far below and a mountain peek directly opposite us on the far side of the valley. For much of the time, vast white clouds of swirling mist engulfed us. From time to time these would miraculously and instantaneously clear, revealing stunning views of snow-capped Alpine peaks which towered high above us, surrounding the peaceful monastery as if cradling it in a protective paternal embrace. On the lower slopes, little hamlets and solitary dwelling places appeared through the mist. And there, far below us lay the city of Tourin, bathed in sunlight, a world away in its bustle and activity.

At night the planets and constellations appeared, their glory unimpeded by the intrusive glare of street lights. The Milky Way cast its pathway across the heavens and we stood, eyes and hearts uplifted, totally caught up in the majesty and wonder of it all. Conscious only of the miracle and fleeting transience of our lives, we felt again that sense of naked reality, which all too seldom stabs its blade of reverent awe into our hearts, reminding us that here we stand, in the holiness of the present moment, each of us just one hair's breadth away from eternity.

Next evening came the storm, magnificent with lightning flashes and resounding thunder! In no time at all, torrents of water gushed from the rooftops, filling water butts and drinking fountains, causing them to spill over into the courtyards. Mountain streams cascaded down the slopes, as if with renewed energy and a fresh resolve to bless and invigorate all surrounding vegetation.

Certainly we were granted a spectacular show, but by the following morning the skies remained heavy and threatening; the rain continued unabated and the monastery lay obscured in a thick grey blanket of mist. At breakfast, I mentioned that I had been hoping for a fine day in which to do a little exploration of the mountain paths. One of my companions jokingly observed that, even with the most fervent of intercessory prayer, it was doubtful that such a transformation in the weather was likely to occur. I had to admit, I shared his pessimism. How wrong we were! Within a couple of hours, Oropa was once again basking in hot sunshine.

Aurelio, our host and organizer of the Anno Domini Multifestival, proved to be the most generous, kind-hearted person. For Dimitri, who had little else to do but to set up his exhibition of paintings, and myself with just two evening performances, this opportunity to relax in such an unusually beautiful setting turned out be nothing other than a holiday. Here, as in Holland, we met with many artists from a variety of European countries. We were able to share our stories, give and receive encouragement, and be enriched by each other's company and artistic gifts.

But there were many other people, apart from the festival goers, visiting the monastery. At weekends, traders set up stalls on the mountain slopes, selling their wares: fruit, vegetables, Italian cheeses, sweetmeats, as well as the many icons depicting Oropa's famous Black Madonna. I formed passing friendships with several people who shared their life-stories with me. Some were facing deep problems and had come to Oropa on personal pilgrimages. I felt privileged when these strangers opened their hearts to me. These were rare moments of apparently chance encounters, our paths randomly crossing for just a few short hours. Who knows what difference these casual meetings make in the greater scheme of things? Perhaps none at all; nevertheless, there is something very special about connecting with people with whom we shall probably never meet again, as long as we live. Here amidst the mountains, priests and pilgrims, trades-people and artists, businessmen and beggars, found themselves bound together in a shared experience: the beauty of Oropa as it nestled so snugly amidst this wild expanse of God's glorious creation. How we wished our family could have been with us; and how strong the desire to share with our loved ones the things that take our breath away.

Our return journey, however, was an entirely different kettle of fish! Our last day in Oropa dawned bright and sunny. I was glad that the UK contingent was scheduled as the final bus-load to depart for the airport. Aurelio, with characteristic generosity, insisted on treating our party to a delicious Italian lunch. Then, at the appointed hour, having waved our farewells, we set off down the winding, often precipitous mountain path towards Tourin, a good ninety minutes' drive away. Poor Dimitri, who is seldom a good traveller when he himself is not at the wheel, soon began to feel desperately ill. Twice during the journey our driver was obliged to stop while Dimitri dived behind the nearest bush! We were all growing increasingly anxious about these delays, particularly for Geoffrey Stevenson, the mime artist, whose flight was due a half-hour or so before ours.

Once at the airport, poor Dimitri fell out of the bus into the nearest gutter, where he collapsed in a semi-conscious heap. Clearly this was something more serious than a bout of travel sickness. The airport doctor was summoned and proceeded to administer his techniques (which included the application of a long and sinister-looking syringe.) Eventually, Dimitri was transported, on a stretcher, to the medical room for further examination whilst I was left to dash about the airport, searching for the appropriate check-in areas and general information desks in the hope that my ailing husband would sufficiently recover in time to catch his flight. As I have already pointed out, I am notorious for having no sense of direction. Many a time I have sent enquiring lorry drivers down one-way or pedestrianized streets, and then, with the realization of my error, been forced to hide behind hedges in order to escape their fury and frustration as they make their retreat. Escalators that were happily rumbling along when I set out on this mission miraculously disappeared as I attempted to retrace my steps. Anxiety and compassion for my sick husband mingled inexplicably with anger. How *dare* Dimitri make such an exhibition of himself!

How *could* he languish so helplessly on the doctor's couch, leaving me to sort out this mess when he knows how perfectly useless I am in these situations!

At last the confounded escalator reappeared, as if out of thin air. Once back in the medical room, I found Dimitri much improved inasmuch as he was now able to stand unaided, although rather shakily, upon his feet. At last the doctor pronounced him well enough to travel, and, although there were only five minutes till take-off, he assured us that he would phone through and stop the airline, informing them of our situation. A mad dash ensued as we attempted to haul our luggage to the check-in point. We could hear our flight number being repeatedly called over the tannoy. In a futile attempt to save time, I squeezed my suitcase through the hand-luggage check-point. This caused a further delay while my scissors and kitchen-knife were confiscated.

What happened next I still find unbelievable. The airport assistants unanimously refused us entry through the gates to board our plane. In spite of repeated exhortations over the loudspeaker, we were turned away on the grounds that the gates had already been closed. In my despair, I tore a strip off the stone-faced woman at the information desk, who calmly told us that our next chance of a flight to Stanstead was in two days time. There was no option but to book these two remaining seats. When I attempted to do so, however, the computer system crashed. There was nothing left to do but wait around until three o'clock the following afternoon, when the Ryanair desk was due to re-open.

It may have been chilly in the mountain mists of Oropa, but here in the busy, polluted airport of Tourin, it was stifling! Fortunately, I had taken a piece of cheese and some bread-sticks from the breakfast table that morning. By midnight I could have died for a cup of tea! At last we found a room for the disabled, where the chairs were slightly less hard than those we had been sitting on all afternoon. We stretched out on the sloping seats and tried to sleep, lulled by the sound of a pneumatic drill which struck up in the early hours, presumably because the noise it produced was considered less intrusive to customers at this time of night.

At 7 a.m., after an uncomfortable night during which we caught only a few odd snatches of sleep, a cleaner appeared, shooing us out of the room with a wave of her duster and a flourish of her broom. A coffee shop was just opening up for the day. Thankfully, we ordered a hot drink and prepared ourselves for a very long wait. All day we hung about that stuffy airport, occasionally dragging ourselves outside for a breath of exhaust-filled air. It seemed that this would quite possibly prove to be the longest twenty-four hours of our lives!

I found a convenient rail in a relatively secluded corner, and as much for my sanity as for any other reason, I whiled away an hour or so doing my barre exercises and stretches.

And so the day dragged on, with Dimitri's condition much improved, but still with serious bouts of vertigo. He was clearly far from well. After hovering about the Ryanair desk for an interminably long time, so as to be first in the queue when opening time came, I once again met up with my sour-faced acquaintance of the previous day. She greeted me with news that the two spare seats which she had spoken of, prior to the computer crashing, were no longer available. There was now no possibility of a flight for another three days. We would need to pay an extra three hundred and eighty euros each, since the longer we were delayed, the higher the cost of a return flight. What a bombshell! Once the initial shock of this news had begun to sink in, we decided to stick around the information desk and continue to hassle every miserable assistant in the hope of a late cancellation.

I am happy to say that this strategy actually paid off. After a very tense interrogation at the end of an extremely long day, the same grim-faced woman announced, in a voice that might equally well have been pronouncing our death sentence, that two seats had become available on the next flight to Stanstead. For one split second I almost felt like hugging her, but quickly checked this impulse when my heart-felt thanks were greeted with a stony glare. Once securely belted into my seat on the aircraft, I could scarcely believe our good fortune. In seemingly no time at all we were back on terra firma, in dear old chilly England. What a relief to be home!

✢ ✢ ✢ ✢ ✢ ✢ ✢ ✢ ✢ ✢ ✢ ✢

As I write, recalling these adventures, I am seated on my bed in the conference centre in Doorn, Holland. It is August 2002, and another CA Festival is underway. Even this trip has not been without its trying moments. Before we left England, Leen La Rivière had emailed to say that Dimitri and I (who were for the first time ever combining our work in a dance presentation with a video and slide projection of Dimitri's paintings) had been allocated a spot in the very first evening concert; the same night as our arrival in Holland. I felt this was most unfair, especially as ours was such a long journey. We had set out at 4 a.m. in order to arrive at Luton Airport in good time. The prospect of dancing in a tired and dishevelled state after hours of travelling, occupied my thoughts all the way to Amsterdam.

On this occasion the trip went remarkably smoothly. We arrived at the pick-up point in Amsterdam and waited…..and waited. An hour later another couple turned up, also from the UK. They were actors from Footprints Theatre Company, and like us, were on their way to the CA Conference. Another hour passed and a whole group of people joined us: story-tellers, singers, musicians and so on. Still no pick-up bus appeared. With the passing of yet another hour we made various attempts at phoning the centre and eventually learnt that a minibus was on its way. By all accounts the traffic in Amsterdam had been unusually bad that day, with all kinds of problems occurring on the roads. By this time, I believe I was the only individual in our company who was feeling relatively pleased about this state of affairs. Almost anything was better than arriving at our destination after more than fourteen hours' travelling, and then being expected to dance! Surely, by now it was impossible to fit in a warm up, a sound check and a rehearsal before the concert?

The minibus appeared at long last. How we cheered! Outside the airport the heavens had opened. Apparently it had been teeming with rain all day. There had been severe storms and flooding. A train had been struck by lightning a few hours earlier, spilling chemicals all over the rail-tracks. Consequently the whole of Amsterdam had been brought to a standstill that day…….and just for me!

For indeed, it seemed that my prayers had been answered! Our spot was postponed until the following Wednesday, and what a great reception we were given! It never ceases to amaze me how much our work is appreciated in Europe, whereas back home, especially in the rural areas of Cornwall, our performances and artwork are frequently met with a much less enthusiastic response.

So much for the adventures of a dancing granny! I hope these tales help to illustrate my earlier point about mountain top experiences.

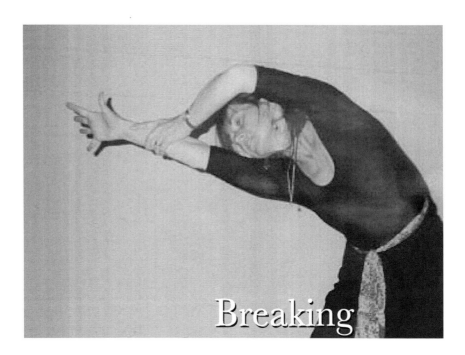

Breaking

Point

And now I come to, perhaps, the very strangest part of my story, which need-less to say, has since become the subject matter for yet another series of dances. I refer once more to those long, shadowy wraiths who so persistently attended me throughout my childhood. One would have expected that, with the dawning of adulthood, such childlike fancies would automatically have disappeared. Not these! Oh I admit, rationally speaking I no longer believed in them, nor in the protection that they supposedly offered. But unlike the fairies of the Never-Never Land, these phantoms refused to die once their credibility had been brought into question. So strong did my ever-growing list of compulsions become, that try as I might to break my habitual slavery to them, I was unable to do so. Any attempt to disregard the rules caused such stress that it was easier to simply comply.

After being set free from night visions, I had attempted to broach the subject of my compulsive behaviour to the Theobalds. But it is not an easy problem to admit to, especially since secrecy plays such an important part in the original pact. At this time, I had never even heard of obsessive compulsive disorder, although a couple of years later I happened to watch a TV programme about a woman who suffered severely from the condition. This was a complete revelation to me...so there were other people in the world whose lives were ruled by these ridiculous compulsions! I was not alone!

I will now quote the rest of the story from my booklet, 'Breaking Point,' which accompanies the dance series by the same title.

✦ ✦ ✦ ✦ ✦ ✦ ✦ ✦ ✦ ✦ ✦ ✦

For most of my life, I have struggled with unreasonable compulsions. As a child I was compelled to do things in certain numbers. For example, if I blinked I was obliged to blink four times, or if I knocked my ankle I would have to make sure that the correct amount of subsequent knocks were administered. All this without anybody noticing of course!

Thoughts also needed to be brought into line, so that even after performing particular strange actions the required amount of times, I invariably had to repeat the whole sequence until I was able to simultaneously think the correct thoughts. Ballet training almost certainly exacerbated the problem since most exercises, enchainments and dance arrangements are set strictly to counts, and each move carefully numbered.

By the time I was married with a young family, constant hand washing had become a major part of my routine. The rules were endless, but dead secret. If I woke in the night I would creep around the children's bedrooms, touching each one on the forehead, feeling like a ghost gliding about on its habitual nocturnal haunts. The hardest part, though, was getting through the bedroom door afterwards, stepping backwards and forwards through the opening as I endeavoured to control my erratic thoughts.

Of course, there were long periods of time when the compulsions grew less, and my habits became so much a part of everyday life that I scarcely noticed them. But during times of anxiety or stress, my obsessions became unbearable. I was quite convinced that this was just an unfortunate, but unavoidable part of my make-up. After the death of my parents, I found my thoughts being taken over to an alarming degree. There were persistent, nagging voices in my head. My mind frequently felt like a battleground.

Ever since experiencing a major deliverance from night horrors in 1990, I have had a desire to help others suffering from similar conditions. When a friend recommended a certain book to me, 'Victory over the Darkness' by Neil Anderson, I bought a copy and began studying it. As I read the case histories of people who had been set free from mental and spiritual strongholds far worse than anything I had ever experienced, I couldn't help wondering if there might possibly be a way out of my obsessive behaviour, if I could but find it.

One night as I lay in bed, I found myself intrigued by a persistent mental picture which seemed to impress itself upon me. The picture was of a part of the inside of my brain, and there, attaching itself to the intricate convolutions, was a cancer. As I focused in on the image, I sensed some fascinating truths being communicated to me.

As cancer cells tend to imitate and take on the form of the normal cells of whichever organ they are invading, so the obsessive compulsive disorder, which I had been host to for so long, had developed alongside me. It had so successfully integrated itself within my personality that I had come to accept that this was simply 'the way I was'. What was revealed to me in that instant, however, was that the disorder was a foreign entity and did not belong there. I asked, not very hopefully, for further guidance, and eventually fell asleep.

I awoke next morning wallowing in the sunshine of a truly wonderful dream; a dream in which I was reunited with my parents and every unresolved problem, every trace of guilt or regret, was dealt with. It was as if Jesus himself had somehow spanned the distance between our worlds and had communicated with us on each other's behalf.

Because of the deep sense of peace instilled within me by this experience, I decided that I would just sit very quietly and meditate for a while, opening myself up to the possible leading of the Spirit. Two scriptures came strongly to mind: firstly, John chapter 16: verse 13 'When He, the Spirit of Truth is come, He will guide you into all truth', and secondly, John chapter 8: verse 32 'You shall know the truth, and the truth will make you free'. I remembered reading in Neil Anderson's book that if we ask the Holy Spirit to lead us to the truth and root cause of a problem, he will do so. I could believe this happened to other people; but to me? Well, I would try.

A few minutes later I was reaching for a pen and paper in order to list the many memories, images, words and dreams that came flooding into my consciousness.

It occurred to me that, as far back as I could remember I had had a sense of being surrounded by a number of long, white beings who had a desire to participate in my life. I slipped back to a day when, at six years old, I had decided to co-operate and allow these apparitions to interact with me.

...........I was in the precise spot; the sun was shining and my brother, Graham, was playing nearby in the stream. I could feel exactly what it was like to be six, and to have the gentle protectiveness of this unusually caring big brother. I had recently come to understand the concept of odd and even numbers, and the pact was that I must do everything in twos and fours. If I submitted myself in total obedience to their rules, these beings would, in turn, offer me protection from all of life's dangers.

As time went by, the chief 'long thing' would sometimes change my number (it was always even) and I lived in terror for a while, in case it had neglected to instruct its companions about the alteration in the rules. I was not at all sure what might happen to me in the event of a slip up like this, and I purposed never to find out!

Before relating any more of my experiences under the Holy Spirit's guidance, it is necessary for me to give some background information about my family.

Two years before I was born, my mother gave birth prematurely to a baby boy, who lived for just four hours. This experience had left her with deep, traumatic scars, and an unutterable sense of regret that she had never been able to hold the child in her arms, for in spite of hearing his cries shortly after the birth, she had been denied any physical contact with him, and was never even granted the opportunity to see the child she had brought into the world.

As I sat meditating that morning, I heard again my sister's voice telling me, as she had done shortly after our mother's death, "The reason you were so special to Mum was because she thought you had the baby's spirit." I recalled, too, that my birthday, March 28th, was the same date as the baby's burial two years earlier, a fact that would have undoubtedly seemed significant to a grieving mother.

125

The night before the child made its premature entrance into the world, my mother, unaware that the pregnancy would not proceed to full-term, had had a strange dream, full of premonitions. In the dream she gave birth to the baby, but was obliged to leave it in a hospital ward. Then her father, already several years dead, appeared, and taking the infant in his arms, disappeared up a winding staircase that led upwards into the heavens. When the funeral took place a week later, my mother recognized the tiny grave as corresponding exactly to the position of the baby's cot in the hospital. Now I began to see that, while on the one hand my mother considered the baby's spirit to be consigned to the care of her deceased father, she also had the vague notion that, two years later, I had become the reincarnation of the child.

The list of dream-memories and associations that continued to flood my mind are seemingly endless, and although essential to the final piecing together of the jigsaw, it is not necessary to relate them all here in detail. I did, however, I find myself puzzling over a vivid mental image which, at first, I couldn't quite make out.

"What can this be?" I pondered, intrigued. The answer came in a flash. The image was a picture of a birth......my birth! Now the fragmented thoughts, impressions and memories began to merge together to form a distinct picture. I had always sensed that in my mother's eyes I had been a replacement, and to some extent a measure of healing for the unresolved trauma. After losing the baby she had suffered several miscarriages and only succeeded in conceiving me with medical help. The picture suggested that, even in the womb, I had been affected by my mother's grief and anxious concern, and it appeared that the confusion of identities between my baby brother and myself had unwittingly invoked some kind of spiritual disorientation.

Now I began to understand the reason for my very special relationship with my brother, Graham. At the time of the baby's death he was just two years old; too young to have any real grasp of what was happening. He was, however, totally caught up in the sense of tragedy that engulfed his mother, in a way which largely escaped our older brother and sister, with their more developed understanding. Since he felt the loss so deeply at this subconscious level, it followed that he would also take upon himself the role of my guardian and protector.

'You shall know the truth and the truth shall set you free'.

How can this be?

When we receive a revelation of truth, there is no alternative but to simply believe it. Feelings don't enter into the equation; it's how we believe that really matters.

The scriptures speak of Christ, *'having disarmed principalities and powers, he made a public spectacle of them, triumphing over them'*(18).

The resurrection, then, is the ultimate triumph over spiritual misalignment and evil. And those who avail themselves of this gift are placed, no matter how unworthily, in a position of grace.

So, in response to this amazing revelation, I thanked God for my salvation, and asked forgiveness for having participated, albeit unwittingly, in a relationship with dubious spiritual powers. I renounced all communication with those ungodly influences and ordered them out of my life.

'Strongholds are mental habit patterns that have been burned into our minds over time, or by the intensity of traumatic experiences.' (Neil Anderson)

In my case those habit patterns had been established over a period of many years, but initially through the intensity of my mother's trauma as it affected me in the womb. Only the Holy Spirit could expose and unravel such a tangle of relational cause and effect. And only Jesus, the redeemer, could offer the solution.

Satanic power invariably originates in the distortion of truth, and in deception. Once the lie is exposed, our minds become free. I knew instantly that I had been released from mental bondage, but of course, the habits took longer to break. Every time I habitually touched something I would think, "I don't have to do that anymore." The sense of freedom was exhilarating.

A few days after my wonderful release I went on a short tour, dancing in the East Midlands. Travelling was normally a somewhat ritualistic matter, so I enjoyed my newfound freedom immensely. When I returned home I embarked on a study of renewing the mind, especially in relation to the persistent voices in my head and the breaking of habits. Naturally speaking this seemed an impossible task, but within a very short time I was getting in control of the situation.

On a couple of occasions something, or someone, attempted to disrupt our peace. Returning home late at night after our Midlands tour, Dimitri and I were very concerned to find a strong smell of burnt wood in the kitchen, but could find no evidence of a fire. Next morning we discovered the charred remains of a kitchen chair outside the back door. When we questioned our son Daniel about it, he replied that he had simply come home the previous evening to find the chair burning! There had been no naked flame anywhere in the house. The chair had stood directly under an indoor washing-line, which had several items of clothing draped over it, airing. Above all this was a wooden ceiling and an open, wooden staircase. It doesn't take much imagination to work out what might have happened to our house if Daniel had not turned up in time!

A day or two later, as I was doing my daily barre exercises, a tremendous crashing and banging made me leap up and rush into the kitchen, expecting to find all my shelves of pots and pans collapsed onto the floor. But nothing was out of place! I returned to my barre, only to have the whole rowdy episode repeat itself a few minutes later.

All this happened in the late summer of 1998. Looking back, I marvel at the freedom I have since come into. It goes without saying that, as a dancer, I had a strong desire to share this liberating experience through my art form; hence the series of three dances entitled Breaking Point. I wanted to engage my audience in the drama, giving an insight into that world of spiritual solicitation, inducement, and finally control of the mind, but culminating in the amazing power of the truth to liberate and heal.

For the first act I have used the discordant music of Vangelis' 'Beaubourg'. My props are, a chair wrapped in white cloth, representing the long white beings of my childhood. Throughout the dance, my combined fascination yet dread of the white ones intensifies, until I am eventually drawn into their power. As I pluck up courage to unwind the cloth, I uncover a long black veil, which becomes my covering and protection.

The movements are often angular and repetitive. I endeavour to conceal my compulsive touching behaviour by pretending to brush my hair aside, or scratching my knee, as you do if you're an OCD sufferer.

I begin the next scene completely shrouded in the black cloth, and flaunt myself around in my new attire like a model on the catwalk. I take on new identity moves. The music, 'JD Food' by Coldcut, is perfect for the piece. There are allusions to a combination of personalities, identities, and bitter, vengeful references to past grievances. As is usual with this kind of spiritual confusion, I slip back and forth from the oppressor to the oppressed.

The key theme to the final dance is, of course, redemption through the revelation of truth. As I mentioned earlier, it was in a dream that the scene was set for my healing. Using Vangelis' music from 'Antarctica', I have tried to capture the feeling of serenity and deep tranquillity that often lingers on after the Holy Spirit's direct intervention through our dreams. The same props are used but their compelling power is diminished. Deep within the folds of the white cloth I discover a long red ribbon, symbolic of the blood of Christ, through whom we receive the revelation of grace and truth. The spell of deception is broken. The power of truth prevails.

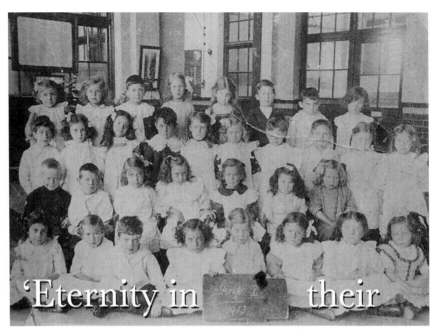

Hearts'

Pupils of Lavender Road School, Enfield. 1913
May Enoch seated front right

Throughout the ages, the hearts of men and women have continued to be stirred by the amazing beauty and mind-boggling complexities of creation, from the humble blade of grass, to the vastness of the solar system, and as we bear witness to these miracles of every day life, many of us are persuaded that such breath-taking precision demands a creator.

Yet these wonders go far beyond what we understand as the physical aspect of creation. Our thoughts and memories, our experiences, emotions and ideas, the energies and spiritual realities which surround us, the unseen laws of the universe, are all equally indicative of intelligent handiwork as are the more tangible aspects of creation. In fact it is often those invisible elements of life that have the greatest impact. Love is surely the most powerful spiritual force; on the other hand, hatred, greed and love of power have consistently wrought havoc throughout history. If mankind is indeed the image-bearer, whose duty it is to 'keep the Garden', it is his God-given calling to steward Earth's resources, to cultivate a life-style of integrity, develop culture, civilization. Creative living is an integral part of what it means to be human, whether it entails the imprinting of 'primitive' images on the surfaces of cave walls, writing a symphony, or playing cowboys and Indians with the kids.

Sadly, the church, which is intended to be a shining light, bearing witness to the love of God and a new revolutionary social order, all too often bows the knee in reverence before the god of consumerism. Day after day we participate in the rape of God's gift to humanity, this jewel of a planet, site of special scientific interest, glorious phenomenon; area of outstanding natural beauty. And while many await the physical manifestation of Antichrist, I suspect that he parades confidently in our midst. If we are honest, much of what we subscribe to: the pursuit of social status, the shops we support, the banks in which we invest our money, all reflect the true nature of our hearts, which, although we often fail to realize it, are all too frequently aligned to this power hungry deity. In its love affair with dualism, the Christian church of today has largely forfeited its ability to function socially, along with its credibility.

Although I could not find it within myself to condemn or unreservedly dismiss any other expression of faith, and in spite of my enormous perplexity concerning many aspects of the biblical narrative, my extraordinary experiences, dreams and visions compel me to describe myself as a Christian. Human beings are naturally religious creatures and, lets face it, we all exercise faith, whether in a religious ideology, a political party or our vitamin pills.

When I was drawn back, so unexpectedly, into the dance scene in 1998, it was with a compelling sense of the need to look into the origins of the faith. Although I had very little understanding of what this entailed at the time, I have since been staggered by my discoveries, which have touched, not so much upon the specifics of religion, as upon the most fundamental, deep-rooted, often primitive yearnings of the human heart.

As a child, I remember my father impressing upon me his deep regard for the wisdom and profundity of the scriptures. He used, as an example, Christ's words as they are recorded in St. Matthew's gospel, *'Whoever has, to him more will be given, but whoever does not have, even that which he appears to have will be taken from him'*(19). Like so many other biblical teachings, this is an age-old principle that still operates on all levels, social as well as spiritual. I have since realized how true my father's words were. The Bible is indeed a remarkable relic of antiquity; a collection of sixty-six books written over a vast time span, using a variety of mediums including symbolism, narrative, historical account, prophecy, poetry, allegory and parable.

Into whichever category one places the creation story it makes little difference to the universal acknowledgement that things are not as they should be. Mankind has failed in his attempt to rule over this beautiful garden, Planet Earth. Basic to all faiths is the concept of 'the way', leading back to a lost age, to an idyllic state of wholeness. The name 'Eden', in the Hebrew language, literally means 'pleasantness'. The story of man's sublime origins in this paradise garden, his temptation, fall, and subsequent banishment into a world of hardship, toil and suffering has, over the centuries, slipped quietly into the realms of ancient mythology. But what if all that vivid, archetypal imagery.... The Tree of Life, The Serpent, The Cherubim, The Flaming Sword, indeed The Garden itself.... were actually essential allegorical truths which act as mirrors, reflecting and revealing the most fundamental elements of humanity? And supposing the Creator of this Earth-Garden, in his omniscience and wisdom, has parabolically woven these many images like clues, pointers, oblique guides, into the very fabric of our being? Half hidden signs which cause us to catch at threads of a subliminal memory buried deep within the universal mind. Maybe the ancient legends, myths, fairy-tales, even our own dreams, might reflect more of reality than most of us ever imagined.

Just as the fruit of the forbidden tree embraces both good and evil, so this bittersweet ambiguity is reflected within the realm of the human soul. The untold beauty of creative gemstones often lies dormant in the 'cellar' of the personality, concealed beneath coverings of guilt, anxiety or shame. Treasure lies shrouded in the shadows. In many of our popular fairy stories, the heroine, that embodiment of supreme virtue, has her rightful inheritance stolen from her and hidden away in some dark, inaccessible, secret place. How like life this is! The thirteenth fairy turns up and casts her spell.(24) Then much of what we deem unacceptable about ourselves is syphoned off, and crammed into the basement along with a pile of gold. Here these shadowy qualities are free to mingle with the gods and goddesses of the underworld. Like dancing phantoms they reappear in the world of our dreams, or perhaps come to greet us in the guise of the fairy-tale characters that we have come to know so well.

.............The frog that retrieves the golden ball from the depths of the well; the lumbering bear with the glimpse of gleaming gold beneath his torn skin; the rats, mice and lizards that are transformed into elegantly prancing horses, or the smartly clothed footmen of Cinderella's coach; that same, beautiful Cinderella who has, for so long, been unjustly consigned to a life of servitude in the basement. All are alive and well today; extensions of the human personality; beings like ourselves, cast out from The Garden of Pleasantness.

Inherent within each of us is a desire for love and acceptance, and above all for our lives to have some kind of significance or meaning. There is a crucial need to re-enter the sacred garden; but let us beware, for many princes perished among the cruel thorns as they sought to awaken the sleeping princess. Not until the appointed time, did the true liberator emerge to deliver the stricken heroine from her death-like sleep.

Typical of most ancient faiths and legends are accounts of dragons, griffins, giants, and all manner of fabulous, often terrifying creatures, which stand guard at the entrances to holy places. Likewise The Sword, The Cherubim, The Garden, The Way, the concept of the need to sacrifice the innocent for the sake of the guilty; these are just a few of the many images that repeatedly crop up in obscure and mysterious guises throughout the scriptures, as well as in the myths and folk-lore of many ancient cultures.

Symbolic of the convergence of law and grace, the revelation of both the Mosaic law (the enforcement of man's alienation) and the tabernacle (the meeting-place of God and man) was given on Mount Horeb, to the accompaniment of searing lightning flashes and thick, billowing clouds of black smoke. The name 'Horeb' is a derivation of the Hebrew word for 'sword', and mysteriously echoes that flaming sword of Eden. *'Mercy and truth have met together; righteousness and peace have kissed each other.'*(20)

It was through the tabernacle (and later the temple) that the ancient Hebrew people received the revelation of the Way to Life. Here was a representation of Eden, essentially prophetic in nature, and symbolic of Christ's earthly body and ministry. Sacrificial rites involving the use of fire and knives were necessary to proceed through each of the entrances, whether gates, doors, or thick veils. And woven into the fabric of these veils of separation from the holiest places, what do we find but those mysterious cherubim once again. Here they stand, in close proximity to exotic flowers, palm trees, pomegranates, and all manner of lush vegetation, reminiscent of the lost gardens of Paradise!

The 'garden enclosed' featured in the Song of Songs, echoes the mystery of love, both human and divine; the scriptural representation of 'the anima', man's union with his deep self and his creator. In fact the entire biblical narrative oozes with a multiplicity of symbolic imagery until finally, Christ, the unblemished Lamb of Passover, is prepared for sacrifice. In total identification with the curse of man, he eats bread with his disciples, sweats blood in Gethsemane, is crowned with thorns by his executioners, and finally dies the ignominious death of a criminal.(21) His tortured body is laid to rest in yet another garden, later to become the setting for his first appearance in resurrected form. But like Psyche's mysterious lover, the face of whom she was forbidden to look upon,(22) the face of Christ remains largely hidden from the world he came to redeem. Let us hold fast to the hope that he will, at the appointed time, emerge to awaken his sleeping bride of lost humanity with the kiss of life.

+ + + + + + + + + + + +

It would appear that the Creator of this world enjoys a good treasure hunt, and is the original author of the cryptic clue! Even Jesus spoke in parables, so as to shroud his teaching in obscurity. But it will be the persistent seekers who will some day have the satisfaction of finding, and those that knock relentlessly who will finally have the door of truth opened to them.(23) Meanwhile, let us allow ourselves to be captivated and enthralled by the magnitude of the divine mystery.

The Glory Hole

Who lives in this dark coal cupboard,
with bars of iron, lock and chain,
secure with dogs, saucer-eyed,
and griffins who guard with winged omnipotence
the entrance to their pit?….
this black abyss where beauty and the gods
play hide-and-seek?
The truant and the misfit,
scorned for inadequacy;
hope, long since vanquished,
whispers still of other worlds
beyond these stifling walls.
Whose hand is this, enclosing mine
in blinding darkness?
A stranger? Yet stranger still
..........familiar;
at whose presence the rusty lock
crumbles into dust.
By dimmest candlelight I follow
as he leads me deeper,
beyond the trap-door,
beneath the cellar;
this basement of my dreams.

Here Cinderella, broom in hand,
tackles the cobwebs, centuries of grime;
a yellow duster, like a golden halo,
tied about crushed curls.
Princess of servitude,
friend of spiders, warty toads,
emptying the rat-trap of rejection;
embraced by creatures of the under-world,
abhorrent to dwellers of the sun-lit uplands.
Those pillars of respectability
whose lot it is to dance in glittering ballrooms,
coyly reclining in the arms, and charms,
of princes.

Further we descend the heaving blackness,
opening doors which creak their way
through haunting memories, long buried
in the earthiness of time.
Here the echo of a child's cry,
there laughter, merriment;
a flash-glimpse of magic,
secret whispering,
then hollow, faceless emptiness.

A bride stands whimpering,
clutching wilted flowers to her breast;
blossoms of youth, long crushed
and faded into wrinkled care;
still anxiously awaiting
the absconding lover;
snatched, stolen or deserted at the crucial hour.
A life that could have been,
perhaps, that should have been;
cast down forever 'midst relentless tyranny
of mocking deities.

Long, long ago,
perhaps before the dawn of memory,
I found a tinder-box
deep in the pocket of my heart;
parched, shrivelled,
with no especial beauty to ignite desire,
yet somehow well belov'd;
a treasure and a breath of hope.
Pulling at the drawstrings
of this pocket-love,
my heart responds with fiery sparks
of sudden flame-ignition.
Recognition.......of you!
long-lost, yet long-awaited
lover of my soul!

Awake now, slumbering Venus!
Shake off your hundred years
of barren, death-like sleep.

Taste once more the sweetness
and the thrill of freedom!
Step out into the highways and the byways
of this underworld.
Embrace the maimed, downtrodden,
the imprisoned and forgotten souls.
Coax forth the shy, reluctant child,
clinging to the skirts of a step-mother
who scornfully exposes all.
Pecked by the mocking-bird
whose shrill screams echo jeering laughter
..........to our shame.
Perching high upon its victim;
its talons searing deep the flesh
of quivering self-abasement.
Yet even she might sing redemption's song,
along with every other jealous thirteenth fairy, (24)
whose thoughtless acts of cruelty
spring from rejection's pain;
the lack of plates being such a feeble excuse!
more akin to lack of compassion!

In the vibrant landscape
of this once invisible world,
so recently fanned into crackling flame
by its own drought,
my shameful, filthy rags
are all at once transformed.
With one fierce blast of searing, holy breath
I stand before you, clothed in purest white.
And far above me,
from the dizzy mountain heights,
The Wild Hunter with a voice of thunder calls,
"Come my child, enter now the life prepared for you.
*You **shall** go to the ball!"*

✢ ✢ ✢ ✢ ✢ ✢ ✢ ✢ ✢ ✢ ✢ ✢ ✢ ✢

'He has made everything beautiful in its time. Also he has put eternity in their hearts, except that no one can find out the work that God does from beginning to end.'(25)

Though many years have spanned the gulf of time since the dawning of my first memories, when the stirring and awakening of the soul wrought impressions that as yet owned no labels, explanations or defining words; when intensity of colour and fascination of texture were experience enough in themselves, and names were neither known nor needed to express them. Yet the magic of life, so pervasive in early childhood, lingers on, albeit concealed for the greater part; occasionally peeping through to give a stab of joy or wonder when one is least expecting it; shattering complacency, obliterating the illusion of our temporal security. Life itself is perhaps a quest for this intangible, illusive quality which refuses to be captured or contained within an idea or equation.

I cannot imagine a time, although I suppose it must come, when I hang up my dancing shoes and abandon forever the desire to captivate the imagination of an audience, while we explore together a realm that can neither be comprehended nor grasped by the intellect. I believe we are, each of us, blessed with an innate awareness of truth and beauty. The ability to stay true to our inborn convictions being so often smothered, almost to the point of extinction, by distorted value systems handed down to us by our predecessors, or by the dominant, cultural word-view of our time.

All of life's experiences, even the more painful ones, somehow have a way of intensifying and endorsing those early persuasions, which were once a part of the very fibre of our being without our ever having learnt them, or even having been truly aware of their presence within us.

A life story is never wholly complete until the life in question draws to a close, but I wait with hopeful expectancy as the future continues to unfold before me. I am forever grateful to my parents for affording me a secure and loving home environment, in which it has been possible for me to discover for myself what would seem to be the priorities of life. This I know they would have given me whether they were rich or poor, for true wealth is of the spirit, even as true freedom is of the mind.

'To me the meanest flower that blows can give thoughts that do often lie too deep for tears'
William Wordsworth

138

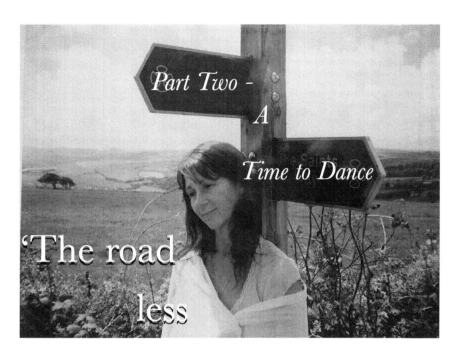

Part Two -
A Time to Dance

'The road less travelled'

Robert Frost

There was once a time when I truly believed that if I were to blow upon a seeding thistle, or dandelion clock, I would send a multitude of fuzzy-headed fairies flying into the wind. Even after realizing the fallacy of this notion, I still chose to pretend that this was the case, and indeed wished it to be so, for the dispersal of such a host of little folk seemed a truly magical affair. Later, with the advent of adulthood, came the perception that nature's diverse methods of propagation are undoubtedly far more amazing than a child's mythical notions of fairyland. For of the countless myriads of seeds that are scattered throughout the countryside, year after year, each one is bursting with the potential for utter transformation; a possible future haven, refuge, feasting ground, for hosts of smaller forms of life; yet how few, in reality, ever chance to undergo that miraculous metamorphosis from tiny coded seed to leafy plant, or mighty tree.

This is true, not only of the proliferation of plants, but also in relation to the human experience. All too frequently exceptional qualities, gifts and talents remain untapped and uncultivated, through lack of encouragement or opportunity. Destiny and potential are two of life's ingredients with which we may all start out, but rarely does any one of us come close to the fulfilment of the latter. And for every hero celebrated in history or folklore, how many unsung heroes now fade into obscurity?

Interwoven throughout our common ancestry is a rich tapestry of creative ingenuity; a vibrant flow of inspiration, revelation and discovery being passed down through the ages. But perhaps, after all, personal recognition is of little importance when compared to the value of a simple life of integrity, and maybe the best inheritance we can leave our children is to teach them to see the miraculous within the humdrum of everyday life; to appreciate the wonder of common things.

It is this sense of the importance of valuing and cherishing the wisdom and skills of our predecessors that spurs me on to write this tribute. And lest my descendants should otherwise be severed from that golden thread of memory which presently links us to an era long since passed, I have taken upon myself the task of relating the life-story of my mother, May Nicholls (née Enoch), whose creative zeal, colourful imagination, and above all her love for dance, made a dramatic impact upon her home community and far beyond. For the enthusiasm with which she sought to fulfil her own dreams, infectious as it was, acted as a catalyst, spilling over into the lives of others, aiding and facilitating them in the discovery and development of their own creative gifts.

✢ ✢ ✢ ✢ ✢ ✢ ✢ ✢ ✢ ✢ ✢ ✢ ✢

May Enoch was born on May 1st 1907; the sixth in what was to become a family of eight children. Her parents, Harry and Emily Enoch, had moved from London's East End to Enfield, in Middlesex, about three years earlier. It had seemed an ideal place to raise their young family, Enfield being, in those days, a market garden town with orchards, open fields, and quiet gravel roads.

The 5 a.m. workmen's train transported the majority of the workforce into London each day, where factories and small businesses flourished. May's father was amongst this multitude of early morning travellers, many of whom like Harry, had first to walk a mile or more from their homes to the railway station. Harry Enoch was a shop-front fitter, a foreman with a firm that carried out development on many of London's larger stores.

Emily, a feather-curler by trade, ran her business from home. Her customers, who came mainly from the surrounding neighbourhood, brought their millinery adornments to her for cleaning and curling. This process involved first steaming the plumes over a simmering kettle, and then beating them dry on a tea towel. Next Emily would work at each individual plume with her special feather-curling knife, deftly applying it to a few strands at a time as she worked her way upwards from the bottom of the feather. The charge for this service was usually sixpence. With ostrich, egret and osprey feathers at the height of fashion, Emily's trade was much in demand.

However, by the time the new baby was six weeks old, this work, as well as most other household duties, had to take second place. May had developed whooping cough and soon became seriously ill. She grew so thin and wasted that Emily found it easier to carry the fragile infant about on a pillow. This she did, day after day, as she walked May out in the fresh air and summer sunshine, often for hours at a time.

Number 42 Hawthorn Grove, where the Enoch family lived, backed on to an enormous playing-field where the local community spent much of their leisure time, often watching the many cricket or football matches which were regularly held there. When relating the story of the baby's illness, my grandmother would invariably conclude with the words, "I wish I had as many farthings as the number of times I walked around that field carrying May on her pillow!"

Life in those days was certainly hard. There was no welfare system or social services to rely upon. A visit from the local doctor was likely to incur expenses which most working-class families were unable to meet. In times of difficulty, friends and neighbours rallied together and did their best to support each other. A strong sense of community spirit prevailed.

As the baby's condition slowly deteriorated, all hope for her recovery began to fade. One bleak evening, while May lay fighting for her life, Mrs.Whitter, Emily's next-door-neighbour, offered her friend some frank, but well-meant advice.

"Put a clean nightdress on her Mrs. Enoch. She won't last the night."

Never having been one to give in lightly, Emily decided to take a gamble. Telling no-one of her intentions she quickly grabbed her purse and ran around to the local chemist. Here she purchased a bottle of Scott's Emulsion, a concoction far too potent to give so young and so feeble an infant.

"Kill or cure!" were Emily's resolute words as May was administered a large dose of the mixture and placed in her cot.

Whether or not all credit should be given to Scott's Emulsion, or whether the divine hand of destiny was at work, is a matter for speculation, but the following three facts are certain. Firstly, that night both mother and baby slept well for the first time in many weeks. Secondly, the child began to make a steady recovery. And finally, ever since that night in the summer of 1907, Scott's Emulsion has been heralded as a life-saver by our family!

How fragile is the web of human life. When one considers the enormous odds against any one of us ever being conceived and born into this world, let alone of being able to sustain life, it seems little short of a miracle that any of us is here at all!

++++++++++++++

My mother was a great storyteller. As a small girl I used to love to hear the much repeated tales of her childhood, often wondering inquisitively what the two sisters, to whom she referred so frequently, actually looked like, little suspecting (for no-one ever told me) that these were my familiar aunties Doris and Elsie. It seemed to me that life in the early part of the twentieth century was filled with a mixture of hard work, wholesome food, sunshine, and long summer days.

How refreshing to live without the menace of the car! A horse-drawn cart clattered along the parched roads in summertime, its driver sprinkling water onto the dry gravel in order to 'lay the dust'. Milkman, coalman, dustman, all relied upon the trusty horse. Until she died in 1958, aged eighty-five years, my Grandmother Enoch regularly left a weekly tip of tuppence for the dustman.

Green living may be a concept of the twenty-first century, which most of us aspire to…but often fail to live up to. During the days of my mother's childhood, people lived an ecological life-style without ever thinking about it. Nothing was wasted. Whatever was not passed down or handed back was used to fuel the boiling copper on washdays. Tradesmen called regularly to collect empty jars in exchange for a ha'penny, or perhaps a toy windmill. Hence the popular music-hall song *'Don't Forget the Ha'penny on the Jam-jar'*.

A woman from Enfield Town trudged the streets, pushing a pram filled with plants. These she would exchange for old or outgrown clothes. Emily regularly offered her refreshment on the doorstep; a welcome cup of tea and a friendly chat. There were rag and bone men calling out for 'old iron', and bartering for all manner of cast off items, offering in exchange goldfishes in jam jars. Like the lighting arrangements of most homes during this period, street lamps were fuelled by gas, and were attended to each evening by the local lamplighter.

Children were expected to help with household chores, especially at weekends when there were shoes to be cleaned, brass to be polished, and extra cakes required to feed the large families, as well as weekend visitors. But there was still ample time for play, and freedom to wander in safety. Children chanted rhymes…*'salt, pepper, mustard, vinegar'*, as they skipped together, a long rope stretched across the dusty road. Other street games included hopscotch, fivestones and hoops; wooden ones for the girls, and iron ones with metal skimmers for the boys. Children were also encouraged to play in the hay in order to help 'turn' it. There were plenty of barns where this commodity was stored, as fodder for the many working horses.

My mother was forever in trouble for her habit of attracting mud and dirt, unlike her younger sister, Elsie, who somehow managed to always stay spotlessly clean. Frequently, the whole family would pack up a large hamper of provisions and walk through the surrounding countryside to Hilly Fields, a favourite picnic spot. In my mother's memory, every summer weekend, and in particular the annual bank holiday at the beginning of August, was invariably blessed with fine weather.

May Day was no exception. What a wonderful day for a birthday! As a small girl, my mother always felt sure that the festivities were especially on her account. Children were dressed in their finest clothes and helped one another to make wreaths and garlands of may blossom with which to decorate the streets and gardens. This grew plentifully all around, as the name Hawthorn Grove suggests. Horses were decked with shining brasses, bells and rosettes; their manes and tails plaited with brightly coloured ribbons.

Empire Day, on May 24th, was also a time of great festivity, particularly during the First World War, when the government of the day was anxious to boost British morale and generate a keen spirit of patriotism. The girls went to school clad in white dresses, decorated with red white and blue flags and artificial flowers made of silk or paper. Emily, who had learned the craft of flower making as a young girl, prepared and supplied endless amounts of these for the local school, as well as for most of the neighbourhood.

Such pride was taken over appearance. It was not unusual for Emily to rise as early as 5 a.m. in order to make new pinafores for her three daughters, with crisp, white frills which needed endless starching and ironing. Frequently, the sisters were granted the opportunity to wallow in self-importance when instructed by their teacher to each stand upon a chair, in order to show off their beautiful new clothes to their less fortunate classmates. All the children were made to parade out into the playground where they were instructed to march around in an orderly fashion and salute the Union Jack.

The playground of Lavender Road School stood literally just a few seconds walk away from the front door of 42 Hawthorn Grove. Over the years a convenient gap had appeared in the school railings, just opposite the house. Through this small space May was just able to squeeze, making her escape at breaktimes, or more especially when she had been forewarned of an essay to be written in afternoon school. She would dash across the road, through the front door, and into the kitchen, where her mother was usually to be found hard at work.

"Mum! We've got to write a composition about the horse. What on earth can I put?" As she continued her household chores Emily would calmly utter all manner of wise sayings. "It is very cruel to cut a horse's tail. This is its only weapon against flies and mosquitoes…" The information was hastily scribbled down and May scampered back to school in relief.

As if she didn't have enough to do already, with her feather-curling work and her eight children to look after, Emily had taken on the job of cooking the seven schoolteachers' dinners each day. This, together with her knack of hob-nobbing with the well-to-do, put her and her family on good terms with the governess and staff, who in those days were considered a race apart. The teachers, stern and austere in their long black dresses, high-necked blouses and button-up boots, looked kindly upon May, in spite of her constant daydreaming and lack of attention.

In one school activity she shone, however. May was unbeatable in athletics. She won all the races, walked off with every sports trophy, and was very soon promoted to the post of netball captain. Her one dread was that of having to write letters to opposing teams, challenging them to matches…but, of course, Emily's help was never far away!

+ + + + + + + + + + + +

The Enochs were an enterprising family. They erected a tent at one end of their small garden from which they sold sweets, homemade ice cream, lemonade and many other delicacies. Emily served the cricketers from the playing field with tea and cold drinks, and May and her sisters helped by cooking all kinds of delicious cakes. In spite of the hard work and long hours, family life was pleasant enough and it seemed that things might well continue in much the same way forever. But with the outbreak of war in 1914, many dramatic changes began to take place. Families were torn apart as fathers and sons were sent off to serve in the armed forces; many of them destined never to return.

During the months that followed, three of May's brothers were called up for military service. Harry, the eldest, was sent to British East Africa, where, after serving in the army for three gruelling years, typhoid almost claimed his life. Having been given up for dead in a remote jungle area, he was miraculously discovered and rescued, and on regaining consciousness, found himself being cared for in a Johannesburg hospital. Harry, like so many young soldiers of that dreadful era, never spoke of these traumas. It was many years later that Emily happened to come across her son's wartime diary, and discovered the truth as she read his account of the many days he had spent lost in the African jungle. Harry had been forced to cut snake bites from his body using his army knife, and in order to survive, had attempted to filter contaminated water for drinking purposes. The entry concluded with the words, "….lay down to die".

Alf, another son, was posted much nearer home, in Aldershot. Due to a slight abnormality of the heart, he was not considered fit for overseas service; whereas George, his seventeen-year-old brother, was forced to suffer the horrors of the French trenches, where he fought as a machine gunner. As a punishment for instinctively ducking to avoid enemy fire, George was appointed the horrifying task of gathering up the dead and wounded: young men and boys whom he had fought along-side in fierce and bloody battles. Like his elder brother, George kept these horrific traumas locked away in his heart, rarely speaking of his wartime experiences.

Families were not permitted to know the whereabouts of their loved ones, but George devised a plan by which he was able to send home coded messages. Initially his family was puzzled by his frequent requests for them to 'look out for Dot', Dot being short for Dorothy, the name of his fiancée. Eventually his younger brother, Wal, noticed that several of the letters were dotted underneath, and when put together spelt the name of Vimy Ridge, George's location in France.

During his final year of over-seas service, George contracted trench fever, which, although very serious, actually proved to be a blessing in disguise. By the time he recovered and had been discharged from hospital, the war was in its final stages. It was during this period of convalescence that George learnt to knit and embroider. The work he turned out was remarkably intricate and finely executed.

And so, miraculously, all three sons returned home in 1919. But who can tell what horrific scars, psychological as well as physical, this generation of young heroes continued to carry throughout their lives? And what of their parents and families, whose thoughts and prayers must always have been with them, never knowing when a telegram bearing ill news might suddenly arrive? Emily's hair turned white during these harrowing years. The wishbone of the 1915 Christmas turkey was kept, along with the Christmas pudding. The latter was boiled up from time to time, and demolished by the returning sons, but the wishbone remains a family keepsake to this day.

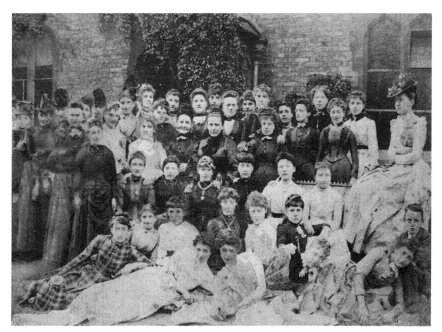

Emily Enoch

Emily aged seventeen lying
centre right, opposite friend Lizzie Banbury
at a church outing in1890

Emily was born on March 23rd 1873, to John and Annie Dunn. Her father was reputed to be 'a thorough gentleman' whose name *could* have been Lorderdale. But as it wasn't, one can only speculate as to why this information was considered of such significance as to be unfailingly mentioned whenever reference was made to my Great-Grandfather Dunn. In keeping with his gentlemanly character, John Dunn held a respectable position of work as a clerk in a customs and excise office, while his wife, Annie, was employed as a bible binder.

The Dunn family consisted of two sons, Alf and Jack, and four daughters, Annie, Ada, Alice and Emily, although I am not sure in what order they arrived. My mother remembered her Uncle Jack bringing home beautifully fashioned, Victorian-style buttons from the button factory where he worked. Her Uncle Alf was employed by Pickfords of London, and every Christmas presented the Enochs with a large turkey and a crate of oranges, which were dubiously described as having 'fallen off the back of a van'.

The eldest daughter, Annie, was reputed to be a great beauty, with large, dark eyes and wonderful curling tresses which were so long that she could sit on them. She, too, worked as a book-binder and was very active in the women's suffrage movement, giving rousing and passionate orations from her soapbox at rallies and demonstrations.

Sadly, Ada died at the age of sixteen from a burst stomach ulcer, after begging her mother to allow her to sample a hot baked potato. She, like Emily, had been a feather-curler by trade.

Poor Alice ended her days in the workhouse where, tragically, she died of melancholia; her husband, mother's Uncle Walter, having allegedly squandered all their money on alcohol. During these times of hardship and extreme poverty, large numbers of old and infirm folk found themselves cast upon this degrading, and often inhuman institution towards the end of their lives. This, too, was the lot of my great-grandmother, Annie Dunn, who spent her final days sitting on her bed, laboriously scrubbing away at an imaginary tub of washing; her husband having died of pneumonia many years earlier; a consequence of his arduous trek to and fro from the workplace in extreme weather conditions, throughout one particularly long wet winter.

My sister and I each have in our possession a brass candlestick with an interesting history. The pair once belonged to Annie Dunn, and quite possibly to her parents before her. Some years after John Dunn's death, my Grandfather Enoch happened to meet his mother-in-law carrying these candlesticks, along with several other belongings, through the London streets towards the local pawnshop. Realizing her intention to pawn these precious possessions, Harry persuaded Annie to allow him to buy them from her, thus keeping the items in the family. My sister's candlestick has a fair-sized dent in it which by all accounts was sustained during a domestic feud. High-spirited Emily allegedly hurled the object at her husband in a fit of rage, thankfully missing her target and smashing into the mantle-piece!

Throughout her childhood, Emily lived with her family in Clerkenwell, in the East End of London, 'close to the home of the poet Robert Browning', so my grandmother always claimed. Browning died in 1889. I cannot imagine a celebrated poet living in such a poor neighbourhood, but since there is usually at least a small grain of truth in these assertions, it is possible that at some stage of his life he had a connection with the area.

As a child, Emily's special friend, and close neighbour, was a girl called Tilly Wood. Tilly came from an extremely poor family, but this misfortune had no apparent ill effect upon her lively charisma and sense of fun. She had an aunt who sang and danced in the London music halls, and Emily was sometimes allowed to accompany her friend to performances, where it was their great joy to be permitted back-stage after the show. Here they mingled with the stars, and even wandered onto the darkened stage, picking up glittering sequins, stray feathers, and other relics of Victorian theatre-land.

The two girls' favourite play area was Bunhill Fields Cemetery, near Old Street, and in particular, perhaps because it resembled a makeshift stage, upon the grave of John Bunyon. Here Tilly would arrange her younger sisters and playmates into theatrical friezes...and woe betide anyone who even so much as blinked an eye-lid unless they were instructed to do so! Tilly also taught her friends to dance the Cancan and the Twist. Under her unyielding eye they zealously practised high kicks and rehearsed many of the popular songs which she had learned from her aunt.

There were flutters of excitement when this fashionable lady drew up in her hansom cab outside Tilly's home. The children were hurriedly sent around to Emily's mother to ask if they might borrow tea cups. Such was their poverty that the family was not in possession of anything as stylish as cups and saucers.

Tilly's father, 'Brush Wood' (so called because he always endeavoured to keep his appearance as immaculate as his spartan income allowed) was an expert at his work, fashioning artificial flowers from crêpe paper; an art which he subsequently passed on to my grandmother, as mentioned earlier, in the account of the May Day festivities. In order to help feed his ever-increasing family (the Woods went on to produce ten children, two of whom died in infancy) 'Brushie' also took an evening job as a waiter, in the infamous Eagle Tavern.

> *'Up and down the city streets,*
> *In and out The Eagle.*
> *That's the way the money goes,*
> *Pop goes the weasel!'*

The more disreputable inhabitants of London's East End were apt to squander their last ha'penny on the purchase of alcohol from this notorious place. 'Pop' being a cockney slang word meaning 'pawn', and the 'weasel' referring to the flat iron used by the tailors; many of whom habitually pawned their work utensils in order to secure beer money.

The Woods and Dunns, however, were devout churchgoers, and regularly attended the local Band of Hope meetings. Every Sunday evening, after the service, the two families gathered together in the Dunns' humble living quarters, where they sang hymns, accompanied by John Dunn on the concertina. The children attended a Sunday school in Old Street. This benevolent establishment, being understandably perturbed at its close proximity to such institutions as The Eagle Tavern and other similar dens of iniquity, encouraged its young members to produce and enact melodramatic scenes, as a means of preaching the gospel and emphasizing moralistic principles. This presented precocious Tilly with a God-given opportunity. With her sisters and friends, she formed a group which she named The Fairy Bell Minstrels. Members were gruellingly put through their paces, and coached for many weeks before their leader allowed them to perform. In one scene, Tilly sang a song about a man who vowed that he would eat his hat if he ever touched a drop of alcohol again. Her sister, Alice, who played the man's wife, appeared in the next scene preparing a stew with the hat when he failed to return home the following night.

It was at a Band of Hope concert that Tilly sang solo for the first time in public. With her rendering of *'Throw Down the Bottle and Never Drink Again'* she brought the house down, instantly winning the hearts of her audience. One gentleman was seen to hurl a bottle of whisky across the room, thus dramatically demonstrating his resolve to never again succumb to the temptations of hard liquor. Tilly, although totally untrained, was a born performer. Unable to hold down any form of conventional employment, her parents reluctantly consented to her performing to the unruly crowds at The Eagle, provided Brushie was present to keep an eye on her. By 1885, at the age of fifteen, she began a steady rise to fame and fortune. Within a very short time she became known as Marie Lloyd, the famous and beloved queen of the music halls.

For many years, Emily and Tilly kept in close contact. Long after she had married and moved to Enfield, Emily still enjoyed occasional nights out at her friend's performances in London. Marie Lloyd, herself, never forgot her humble beginnings, and always made a point of maintaining her contact with the poor and underprivileged. Her generosity was limitless, and one year she bought every child in her home town a pair of warm winter boots. If she ever happened to catch sight of Emily, in the street or queuing for tickets at the box-office, she would draw up in her cab, and with a hearty, "Whatch-yer Em!" together they would strike up a conversation about old times.

When relating these tales to us, my grandmother always emphatically denied that her friend was in any way flighty or promiscuous. (Having read a couple of Marie Lloyd's biographies I find this increasingly difficult to believe, but out of respect for my grandmother I must take her at her word!) This reputation resulted from a façade, an impression that was created as she played to her audience. In reality, Emily insisted, Marie Lloyd was as respectable and upright as the poor, but God-fearing family she came from.

It is my belief that this influence upon Emily Dunn's life, her captivation and love of music, dance and theatre, has somehow permeated the genes of her descendants, many of whom seem set to continue in the pursuit of that same creative magic for many years to come.

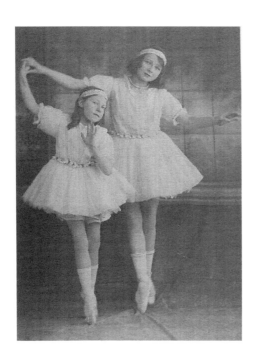

First

Steps

Elsie and May circa 1919

Nowadays it is not so very unusual for little girls to attend dancing lessons. However, this was far from the case during my mother's childhood. British ballet was then very much in its infancy, and precious few young people were ever fortunate enough to become acquainted with its techniques. So it was with a great sense of wonder and excitement that May and her little sister, Elsie, were escorted by their mother to Gamba of Dean Street, in the West End of London, to buy ballet shoes.

The following week, under conditions of extreme secrecy (on no account were they to tell their father) the girls were taken to The Violet Minnafie School of Dancing for their first ballet lesson. May, being the elder of the two, was under strict instructions to tell her teacher (should she be asked) that Elsie was seven years old, this being the age from which pupils were admitted into the school. In fact she was short of this by a few weeks (give or take the odd month!) But I am sure that Miss Minnafie, who obviously had a living to make and a reputation to uphold, would not have quibbled over this minor discrepancy once she discovered what talent had been sent her way!

Both girls took to dancing like ducks, or perhaps I should say swans, to water, and very soon began to excel in this exciting new accomplishment. They swaggered off to their weekly lesson, pointe shoes in hand, much to the envy of many of their peers. These secret lessons continued for a little over two years. Then, in 1919, Harry returned from overseas military service. As a 'welcome home' surprise May and Elsie, still sworn to secrecy, were dressed in full Irish costume, cleverly made for them by their mother, and sent into the living room at the appropriate moment to perform an Irish jig before their astonished family, ending as instructed with the chant, *"Now Harry's come home from Africa!"*

I am sure that Emily waited with confident anticipation for her husband's reaction. He was both amazed and delighted, and apparently not at all put out at having been kept in the dark for so long! From this moment on he gave his full support to his two younger daughters' education in dance; Miss Minnafie also benefiting from his enthusiasm in-as-much as she was never without elaborately constructed scenery for her concerts.

By the time she was fourteen years old, May had generated a following of enthusiastic youngsters, who met regularly for free dance practices in the recreation field behind her house. A born organizer, May arranged a variety of scenes, dances, solos and duets for these young prodigies, as well as for herself and Elsie. Emily jokingly named the group The Dusthole Fairies, as their rehearsals took place close to the spot where the rubbish bins stood. When an adequate repertoire had been devised….The Toy Shop, Le Carnaval, Butterflies and so on, it was announced that a concert was to take place the following Saturday afternoon in the large playing-field at the back of Hawthorn Grove.

On the appointed day, benches were borrowed and collected from the nearby church hall; the wind-up gramophone, with its long horn, was given a thorough checking over, and Emily and the girls busied themselves with the preparation of refreshments. By all accounts several relatives also turned up for the occasion. May's Aunt Nell happened to be standing by the bay window in the Enoch's living-room, which overlooked the approach to Hawthorn Grove. From the kitchen, Emily heard her sister-in-law calling excitedly, "Come and look at this, Em!" And there, streaming along the road were crowds of local people, all making their way to the concert. The cricket and tennis players also abandoned their matches for the day in favour of an afternoon's live entertainment.

The concert was a huge success. Free homemade lemonade was distributed (cunningly served in thick-bottomed glasses so as to create the illusion of extra generous servings) and a collection was taken up which amounted to a grand total of five pounds, five shillings and fourpence, which in 1921 was a considerably substantial sum. Harry Enoch, notorious for his generosity, insisted that the proceeds be donated to the Enfield Cottage Hospital.

Needless to say, the hospital proprietor and staff were delighted with this unexpected gift. The donations, as well as the concerts, became a regular feature of Enfield community life. It was not long before May was being called upon to produce shows in aid of church and hospital funds, garden fêtes, and all manner of local charities.

Backdrop to
The Ballets Russes

In 1909, following his highly successful introduction of Russian painting (and later opera) to the elite of Parisian society, the impresario, Sergei Diaghilev, turned with enthusiasm to his next project: the revelation of the wonders of the Russian ballet to the Western world.

During his time as artistic director to the Maryinsky Theatre of St. Petersburg, Diaghilev had made the acquaintance of a growing number of young, exceptionally gifted dancers and choreographers, who desperately needed the opportunity to expand beyond the limitations and rigidity of the Russian Imperial Ballet. Artists such as Vaslav Nijinsky, Tamara Karsavina, Lydia Lopokova, and dancer/choreographer Mikhail Fokine, who, but for his innovative spirit and desire to experiment beyond the perimeters of tradition, would undoubtedly have replaced the legendary but aged Petipa as permanent choreographer to the Maryinsky Theatre. Fokine, under Diaghilev's cultivating influence, became the creator of many popular and much-loved ballets including Les Sylphides, Le Spectre de la Rose, Petrouchka, The Firebird, Schéhérazade.

These prodigies Diaghilev gathered under his wing, eventually to form The Ballets Russes, along with other currently little known artists, including the designer Léon Bakst, the painters Alexandre Benois and Pablo Picasso, and the young musician/composer, Igor Stravinsky, who, thanks to Diaghilev's encouragement and support, eventually went on to produce many of the revolutionary masterpieces and musical scores which were to inspire Fokine, and later Nijinsky, in the creation of new, ground-breaking ballets.

Many times during its turbulent history, The Ballets Russes came perilously close to bankruptcy, but with Diaghilev's vision and dogged determination, not to mention his influential connections with members of the aristocracy, the company always succeeded in pulling through. Throughout this extraordinary era many other emerging artists were detected by the great impresario and drawn into this unique amalgamation of creative brilliance: Matisse, Massine, Rambert, Markova, Ballanchine, Satie, Ravel, to name but a few. Even the legendary Anna Pavlova danced for Diaghilev before forming her own company here in England in 1911.

And so it happened that Paris, in the spring of 1909, was overwhelmed by its first encounter with the Russian Ballet. The following year, with Diaghilev's first Covent Garden season, London audiences, too, were bowled over by the unparalleled virtuosity of this remarkable new company, the effects of which were to influence and totally transform the future of ballet world-wide.

✦ ✦ ✦ ✦ ✦ ✦ ✦ ✦ ✦ ✦ ✦ ✦ ✦

The Enochs were among the few working class families ever fortunate enough to witness the wonders of The Ballets Russes during its UK seasons. Working, as he did, in the centre of London, Harry Enoch would listen eagerly for news of the company's imminent arrival. There was great excitement when, on the appointed Saturday, Emily and the girls caught the train into town and made their way to the West End, where they joined the long queue outside the theatre box office. On these occasions Harry, who worked a half day on Saturdays, would arrange to meet his wife and daughters straight from work, by which time several hours had already been spent queuing. The long wait was not so very tedious, however. There was plenty of street entertainment, with buskers, singers and jugglers, as well as street traders pushing their wheelbarrows filled with hot chestnuts to nibble.

At long last the theatre doors opened and the crowds surged forward. There followed a frantic race to climb the seemingly endless flights of stairs that led to the upper circle, or 'gods'. Harry, a hefty man, would call to the girls to run on ahead and find seats, while he and Emily followed eagerly from behind, puffing and panting with the extra exertion.

There they sat, amongst the privileged few, for in those days ballet audiences consisted mainly of professional people, intellectuals, ballet teachers, and those who held exalted positions in the world of theatre and the arts. Enthralled, May and Elsie fell captive to the magic of Pavlova as she danced her famous roles: The Dying Swan, The Dragonfly, Columbine and many others. They witnessed the flawless technique and impeccable genius of Nijinsky, their eyes shining in wonder and disbelief at his apparent ability to hover in mid-air. They were present at Drury Lane Theatre when he executed his famous leap through the open window of the stage set, crossing the length of the entire stage in one enormous bound, as he partnered Karsavina in Le Spectre de la Rose.

The two girls felt themselves transported into another world, a magical world of artistry, stunning beauty and fantasy. During the interval, the sisters chattered excitedly to each other, imagining themselves being invited on stage to demonstrate their ability to execute all kinds of intricate steps and enchainments. May, especially, was aware of the enormous privilege of being present at these unique performances, and with the quickening of her own creative spirit, inspiration for new projects began to emerge....much to the delight of The Dusthole Fairies!

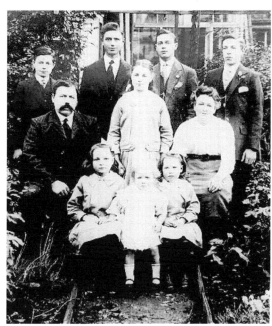

A hard-knock life

The Enoch family in 1919
Back- left to right, Wal, Harry, Alf, George.
Centre- Harry, Doris, Emily. Front- May, Les, Elsie.

In the relatively small family circles of the present day, it is not unusual for the youngest member to enjoy a good deal of attention from indulgent parents and doting older brothers and sisters. But when one considers the tremendously hard work involved in caring for large numbers of children, especially without the aid of modern domestic appliances, it is perhaps little wonder that, during the period in question, the baby of the family invariably found itself considerably less than over-indulged.

This was certainly the experience of May's youngest brother, Leslie John, who was born in 1913. It was unusual for trained midwives, or indeed anyone with medical expertise, to be called upon to assist in anything other than extremely difficult births, but on this occasion the local doctor did put in an appearance shortly after the safe arrival of the child.

"So Mrs. Enoch, you have a fine son! What had you been hoping for this time, a boy or a girl?"

"Neither!" was the decisive reply.

Although May was only six years his senior, she very quickly took her small brother under her wing, acting as a second little mother to him and protecting him from the taunts and teasing of the older siblings. The emotional needs of the very young were not given much consideration during these times, and so, being easy targets, small children frequently became the object of ridicule and disparagement.

Fortunately Harry, the eldest son, had a kind-hearted disposition and often did his best to relieve his sisters and younger brother from humiliation. It was while walking home late one evening that Harry happened to meet his distraught mother, wheeling a screaming baby Les along the road in his pram.

"Wherever are you going at this time of night, Mother?" he asked, shouting in order to be heard above the hullabaloo.

"I'm on my way to the river to drown this little b….!" came the frenzied reply.

Taking the shrieking infant from his mother, Harry eventually succeeded in pacifying the child, and the three were soon able to return home in a state of relative calm. Perhaps we, like Harry, must give Emily the benefit of the doubt in assuming that, in this case, her intentions were not wholly criminal!

My Uncle Les grew up to become a kind, gentle, hard-working man. He served in the Royal Air Force during the Second World War and on his return, studied horticulture. He was later promoted to the position of head gardener for the Enfield area hospitals. Uncle Les remained forever grateful to my mother for her affectionate protection, and I am sure his gratitude also extended to Uncle Harry, for rescuing him from a watery grave!

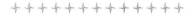

Wal (Walter) Enoch was unlike his eldest brother, inasmuch as he failed to emanate such an abundance of warm-hearted affection towards his younger siblings. Instead, he took great delight in teasing and tormenting them. Perhaps in an attempt to alleviate the distress inflicted upon these unfortunate little ones by the relentless provocations of this particularly tiresome big brother, Wal's parents endeavoured to channel their son's surplus energy into something rather more creative. As he already showed considerable promise at the piano, he was presented with a violin and promptly packed off to music lessons. But Wal vehemently hated these lessons, which came to an abrupt end when he broke his arm. Once the arm mended, Wal vowed to keep well clear of his music teacher. Instead he taught himself to play both instruments solely by ear, proving himself to be an extraordinarily gifted musician. This was to prove invaluable in later years, especially in the production of May's concerts.

Presumably in order to create yet another outlet for his relentless energy, Wal took to riding (and frequently crashing) motorbikes. Following one very serious accident, he was admitted to Enfield General Hospital, where he remained in a coma for more than three weeks. Kind-hearted Harry, with great brotherly concern, arranged for the local church choir to assemble in the hospital ward around Wal's bed, from whence they proceeded to serenade him with hymns. During the singing, Wal slowly began to regain consciousness. Seeing himself surrounded by this heavenly ensemble, he immediately assumed that he had died, and had somehow succeeded in passing through those pearly gates to the Celestial City….in spite of all the torment he had inflicted upon his family in his previous life!

Wal eventually made a complete recovery, only to crash his motorbike yet again. However, on this occasion he remained fully conscious throughout the whole experience. He was so horrified that he vowed never to ride again. Presumably a great relief to his long-suffering parents!

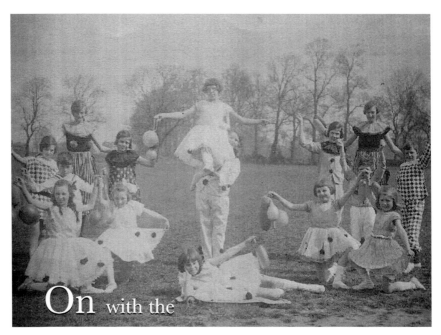

On with the
show

'The Dusthole Fairies' in 'The Toyshop'. May and Elsie in centre lift.

As each of the Enoch girls neared school-leaving age, there was much deliberation as to what their future lines of employment might be. Doris, the eldest, found work in a factory, making lampshades. Elsie finally gave up her dancing and went to London where she trained as a dressmaker. She was very gifted in her work and after qualifying, went on to receive commissions from royalty.

In 1923, at the age of sixteen, May left The Violette Minnafie School and was accepted as a full-time professional student at The Briscoe School of Dancing. Here she trained for six days a week over the course of the next twelve months. In addition to this, and by way of earning her keep, she shared the workload with her mother in the home, cooking, cleaning and generally keeping house for all the family. The following year she was sent to audition for a part in a production at The Chelsea Palace Theatre, in London. The person conducting the audition was a certain Miss Fairburn, a well-known figure in the dance world at that time, who terrified May by her austere manner.

It was not long before May was singled out and ordered to execute eight cobbles, a difficult step in Russian dancing which requires enormous strength and panache. May responded effortlessly to Miss Fairburn's command.

"Now do sixteen!" was the stern response; May obliged; "Now thirty-two!" Once again May obediently complied with the request; "Now high cabrioles!"

If May's demonstration was in any way pleasing to the uncompromising Miss Fairburn, there was nothing in her voice that betrayed her approval as she shouted her final command.

"Come here!"

May looked around hopefully at the other dancers. Perhaps this terrifying lady was not addressing her after all. Maybe some other victim was being singled out. But no such luck! As if summoned to her execution May walked in fear and trepidation towards Miss Fairburn's desk. Again the stern voice boomed in her ear. "May Enoch, you are a very good all-round dancer. You have been chosen for the leading role in Tchaikovsky's Trepak."

It was during this season at The Chelsea Palace Theatre that May decided once and for all time that her career choice lay, not so much in performance, but in teaching and producing her own shows. She was essentially a homebird and the prospect of an uncertain future, in what appeared to be a rather frightening and unpredictable environment, did not really appeal to her.

And so the following year, May, now aged seventeen, began to prepare for a new venture. She made enquiries, and discovered that the local Sunday school hall was available for hire at a reasonable cost. Her father made her a fine set of portable ballet barres, and Emily helped to write the advertisement for the Enfield Gazette, 'The Dancing child is a happy child. Why not let yours learn now!' This produced a good response. May began with ten pupils at a cost of one shilling per lesson. She also gave private tuition to children of wealthier families. Little by little the numbers in the classes increased until she found herself running a thriving dance school with over one hundred pupils.

Of course, May already enjoyed an excellent reputation for producing shows in an unofficial capacity. It was not long before she was being approached by all kinds of organizations seeking help with their entertainment arrangements. This was the era of the first sound movies. Picture palaces were flourishing everywhere. An evening's programme consisted of two films, with an interlude of about thirty minutes in between. May was asked by several cinema managers to provide entertainment during the break. To do this on a regular basis required a full and varied repertoire, as well as a great deal of hard work.

But there were also full-scale concerts to organize. Taking a bus-ride into Enfield Town shortly before her first official production, May was shocked to see her name splashed across huge billboards, advertising her forth-coming show. She had certainly not counted on this kind of exposure, and it filled her with trepidation. But there could be no turning back at this late stage. The show, as they say, must go on!

+ + + + + + + + + + + +

At last the day of the concert arrived; family and friends pulled together in a mutual desire to make the event a success. While May busied herself backstage supervising her pupils, Emily bustled about beside her with an air of great importance.

"There are crowds of people outside," she announced. "The queues reach right to the end of the street. Goodness knows how we're going to fit everybody in!" But fit them in they did! Extra benches were fetched, and children crammed themselves together on window sills. No restrictive health and safety regulations in those days!

"What's Dad like?" May asked her mother anxiously. "How's he taking it?" Emily peeped through the side-curtains into the auditorium where her husband was graciously ushering the elderly folk to the front seats, which he had taken care to reserve for them. "He's as proud as a peacock!" she assured her daughter, with more than a hint of pride in her own voice.

Indeed he was, and how Harry worked to ensure the success of this and all subsequent productions! Using his carpentry skills he made wings for the oth-

erwise bare stages, produced all manner of scenery, and constructed an elaborate proscenium arch. Nothing was too much trouble for him. He arranged
the hiring and use of footlights; helped with advertising, the printing of tickets, and was always to be found on performance evenings tending to the com-
forts of the audience.

Indeed, the whole family, as well as many eager friends and neighbours, regularly contributed their services on these occasions, offering their various skills
and abilities with great willingness. All were pleased to feel, in some small way,
a part of the production team. During this period, before the advent of TV,
video, CD or DVD players, live entertainment was highly valued, and was
always well supported by the local community.

Elsie, with her dressmaking expertise, designed and created the most elaborate
costumes, often with the help of Emily. May's friend, Mara Payne, shared with
Doris the job of playing for the concerts. Both were accomplished pianists.
Even Wal eventually consented to being roped in to arranging and adapting
all the live music to the specific requirements.

Other willing volunteers involved themselves in arrangements for décor, the box
office, seating and front of house administration, as well as acting as ushers to
the general public on performance nights. Every detail received due attention,
and each willing helper was inevitably drawn into the magic of theatre.

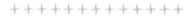

May's confidence and popularity continued to blossom as the demand for her
work increased. She received invitations to dance at The Edmonton Empire,
once a London music hall, now run by Bernstein along with a whole chain of
London theatres and picture palaces. Here May and her pupils performed to
packed houses, receiving tumultuous applause and praise-worthy press
reports.

Amongst her greatest achievements was The Gipsy Beggar, a story depicting
a young girl, played by May herself, aged just seventeen, who is forced to make
her meagre living as a fortune-teller. However, when the foretelling of unre-

quited love fails to please her master, she is turned out of her home and compelled to dance herself to the grave. Set to Lizt's Hungarian Rhapsody, this powerful combination of dance and drama proved an outstanding success.

Later, in 1927, May choreographed and staged another hugely successful work, entitled The Slave Market. In an exotic Eastern setting, this story portrayed the lot of a downtrodden slave-girl who suffers ill-treatment and abuse at the hands of a rich taskmaster. Katelbey's music, *In a Persian Market*, proved the perfect choice for the piece. Colourful stage sets and flamboyant costumes, including a genuine rhino-tail whip (a relic of Harry's adventures in Africa) all contributed to evoke a captivating atmosphere of authenticity.

How ironic that the little girl who had previously found such difficulty in composing an essay for her English teacher should, of her own volition, engage herself in creating such stories! And not only so, but also in setting the scenes to music, casting parts, she herself dancing in and directing the whole venture, and finally presenting the completed works before delighted audiences!

+ + + + + + + + + + + +

With the ever-increasing demand for her work, it became essential for May to constantly devise new and original ideas for adaptation into dance and dramatic arrangements. Determined to keep informed of all the latest dance styles, she began taking lessons herself in tap and ballroom dancing, travelling to London every week in order to brush up on the fox-trot, waltz, quick-step, and that most innovative and flamboyant of dances, the tango. It was not long before The Mae Enoch School of Dancing was offering tuition in an abundant variety of dance styles.

Undoubtedly, May became the apple of many a young man's eye, and it was at these ballroom dancing sessions, during the spring of 1925, that she met her future husband, William Nicholls. Bill, as he was generally known, was a handsome, rather quiet person, and a deep thinker. He had suffered much hardship during the course of his young life, following the death of his father in 1919. At the age of thirteen he had been obliged to leave school and, together with his two elder sisters, had adopted the role of bread-winner for the family. He too lived in Enfield, where he worked as a dental technician. The couple soon began planning a future together, saving from their earnings week by week for the deposit on a house. To be married with a home of her own spelt freedom to May, whose work in the Enoch household weighed increasingly heavily upon her, sapping her energy and restricting her creativity.

The wedding took place on Easter Monday, April 21st 1930, at Jesus Church, Forty Hill, Enfield. Since both were highly respected members of the community, the event caused a considerable stir. Crowds of well-wishers turned up at the church, in addition to the many friends and family members who were, of course, invited. May was clad in a dress of mirror velvet, designed for her by her sister Elsie, who was now employed by Dickens and Jones of London and receiving commissions from the Princess Royal, as well as creating saris for a number of Indian princesses. Elsie also made the bridesmaids' dresses; for herself, Harry's fiancée Marjorie, and three of May's pupils. They carried bouquets of yellow tulips and grape hyacinths, while the bride's flowers consisted of cream-coloured tea-roses and lilies-of-the-valley. May, herself, made the wedding cake, an impressive affair comprising three tiers, elaborately iced and decorated.

After their honeymoon, spent in Porlock, Somerset, May was eager to return to Enfield and move into her new home. Released at last from the workload of 42 Hawthorn Grove, she settled happily into married life. The many years of working alongside her mother had resulted in her becoming an excellent cook and proficient homemaker. Bill was, as always, highly supportive of her dancing, and together they planned many new productions. Evidently, news of the excellent quality of May's work had spread well beyond the bounds of her home town, for The Italia Conti Stage School, of London, developed an annoying habit of sending talent scouts to her shows, and on several occasions succeeded in luring away some of her most promising pupils.

In September 1931 my sister, Diana, was born; the apple of Enfield's eye! By the time she was three years old Diana was known as 'Enfield's Little Shirley Temple', singing and dancing in all the shows with uninhibited abandon. Even when, four years later in 1935, my brother Barrie came along, May's dance work continued unabated. Having small children of her own simply inspired her to include them in her productions. Barrie made his début, somewhat reluctantly, at around two years old. His lack of enthusiasm stemmed, not so much from the prospect of performing, but was chiefly due to the injustice of being made to wear a prickly suit. Nor was he best pleased to see his mother attempting to prompt him from the wings.

"Don'ch, Mummy! Don'ch!" he responded indignantly, inadvertently sending the audience into fits of laughter.

And so, the Nicholls family continued to lead full and really rather exciting lives. They moved into a larger house, where May was able to hold classes on the premises and also take in lodgers. One of these tenants was a gentleman by the name of Mr. Chaimberlain, a name that evidently inspired a good deal of confusion in little Barrie's mind........Could it really be that the Prime Minister was renting the room upstairs?

'To everything there is a season,
A time and a purpose under heaven.
A time to weep, and a time to laugh;
A time to mourn, and a time to dance.
A time to love, and a time to hate;
A time of war, and a time of peace.'(26)

The outbreak of World War Two, in 1939, brought abrupt and dramatic changes to the lives of many people, particularly those dwelling in or around the London area. Nights were often fraught with anxiety, and sleep disturbed by frequent air-raids. Food and clothing were rationed. The reality of the fragility of human life was ever present in people's minds, and as time passed, few remained unaffected by the loss of friends, neighbours, or loved ones. My family miraculously escaped unhurt when a bomb exploded just a few feet from their house. The wooden sign advertising *'Mae Enoch - Dancing Classes'* was chipped in the blast, but thankfully, no real damage occurred.

My father was not called up for military service, being above the required age. He continued in his dental work and contributed on a voluntary basis as a fire-watcher. With the black-outs came the closure of all cinemas and theatres. May continued to teach, but numbers dwindled as the incentive of working towards performances was inevitably lost.

In December 1941 my brother, Graham, was born, entering the world at a time of tension, conflict and uncertainty. In spite of the fact that she was suffering from fatigue, and had a growing desire to be at home with her family, May felt obliged to return to her teaching as soon as possible.

Interminably, the war dragged on, taking its toll on the lives and well-being of all who endured those troubled years. Anxiety and exhaustion were slowly undermining my mother's health and when, two years later a forth child was born prematurely, and subsequently died, she became engulfed in a grief that was almost impossible to bear. Perhaps it was this sense of loss which caused my parents to consider a complete turn-about in the direction of their lives.

By the time I appeared on the scene, in March 1946, the war was over, and the family was contemplating the possibility of embarking upon an entirely new life. However, it was to take another eighteen months before all plans slotted into place, and we were finally able to move away from the pressures of suburban life, to the comparative peace and tranquillity of South Devon. Here it seemed impractical for my mother to establish any further dancing schools. Instead she undertook the running of a large guest house at Bigbury-on-sea. My father also helped with the administration of this new enterprise during their first summer season. However, establishing a business of this kind so soon after war proved difficult, and the move turned out to be pretty much a financial disaster. Before long my father found work with a dentist in St. Austell, Cornwall. The considerable distance made it necessary for him to lodge away from home during the week, returning to Bigbury at weekends. Although I was only two years old at the time, I remember the excitement of seeing him turn up on a Friday evening, usually with a packet of plasticine, a pot of bubbles, or some other little surprise for Graham and myself.

My mother was so busy running the guest house that Diana, now seventeen years old, spent most of her time taking care of me. I remember wandering with her across the vast expanse of the deserted beach on a summer's evening, discovering the ripples in the sand, left behind by the retreating tide. I was taken each day to visit a horse named Twilight, who lived in a field close to our house, so it is perhaps little wonder that I recall being hoisted aloft a five-bar gate and stroking the velvet nose which so obligingly thrust itself into my small hand.

Within a short time of my father taking the job in Cornwall, it was decided that the rest of the family should move down to join him. This exodus occurred in January 1949, and, biased as I undoubtedly am, I shall be forever grateful for this turn of events. I can think of no better place to spend one's childhood. We youngsters were blessed with freedom to wander and play in safety, surrounded by farms, fields and woodlands, as well as by the most glorious coastline with its unspoilt beauty, safe beaches and gentle sea.

In contrast, my mother suffered something of a culture shock, having been uprooted from her home-town where her work and talents had been so widely appreciated. She now found herself immersed in the depths of the Cornish countryside, surrounded by folk of a seemingly alien culture. People who, apparently, had no great interest in the performing arts, and had probably never even heard of Pavlova, Nijinsky, or Diaghilev's Ballets Russes!

However, the artistic drive and love of theatre continues to permeate our family line. Thanks to my parents' support, hard work and unwavering encouragement, many of their offspring have become flourishing musicians, singers, artists and creative thinkers. The enchantment which captivated the imagination of the child, Emily Dunn, her friendship with Marie Lloyd, and their association with the London music halls, continues to vibrate in the hearts of her descendents, three and four generations down the line.

Talk about holes in the ozone! What an enormous vacuum there would have been in our world if The Almighty had not chosen, against all odds, for that tiny baby to recover from whooping cough, and live out her life so richly and so creatively. And what a blessing that Emily, with her dogged determination, was prepared to take a gamble. May we, her descendants, be forever grateful to the amazing power of Scott's Emulsion!

Life is more than the pursuit of wealth,
Or even of happiness.
It is wider than the boundaries
That extend beyond birth and the grave;
Greater even than the elusive magic
Which pervades our childhood;
The beauty of creation, music, art.

For these would seem but a foretaste,
Given to instill in us a certain wistfulness;
A yearning for that greater mystery
Of which all that we love and cherish
Is but a shadow, a signpost,
Which leads us on, beyond ourselves;
Beyond the visible and transitory,
Onwards and upwards
Towards the One who is Himself
Reality and Life.

References

(1)   Psalm 139: v 14

(2)   William Wordsworth - Ode - Intimations of Immortality

(3)   The Beatles – Fixing a Hole Where the Rain Gets In
       Sergeant Pepper's Lonely Hearts Club

(4)   The Beatles – Strawberry Fields

(5)   The Beatles - Lucy in the Sky With Diamonds

(6)   The Beatles – Eleanor Rigby

(7)   Friedrich Neitzche – Thus Spake Zarathustra

(8)   Bob Dylan - Man of Peace

(9)   Calvin Seirveldt - Rainbows for the Fallen World

(10)   Hebrews Ch 13: v 2

(11)   Bob Dylan - Sweetheart like You

(12)   Psalm 133: vs 2-3

(13)   Psalm 19: v 1

(14)   Proverbs Ch 8: vs 1-2 & 22-31

(15)   Psalm 42: v 7

(16)   Genesis Ch 25: v 23

(17)   Ezekiel Ch 37: vs 1-14

(18)   Colossians Ch 2: v 15

(19)   Matthew Ch 25: v 29

(20)   Psalm 85: v 10

(21)   Genesis Ch 3: vs 17-19

(22)   Cupid and Psyche (Roman myth)

(23)   Matthew Ch 7: v 7

(24)   The thirteenth fairy in the tale 'Sleeping Beauty', who cast a spell over the palace
       because she was not invited to the princess's christening party on the grounds that
       there were not enough plates.

25)   Ecclesiastes Ch 3: v 11

(26)   Ecclesiastes Ch 3: v 1, 4, 8